POLISHING
THE
MIRROR

OTHER BOOKS BY RAM DASS

RAM DASS AUDIO FROM SOUNDS TRUE

POLISHING THE MIRROR

How to Live from Your Spiritual Heart

Ram Dass

with Rameshwar Das

Conceived by Janaki Sandy Gaal

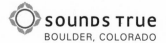

SOUNDS TRUE
BOULDER, COLORADO

Sounds True

Boulder, CO 80306

© 2013, 2014 by the Love Serve Remember Foundation

SOUNDS TRUE is a trademark of Sounds True, Inc. All rights reserved. No part of this book may be used or reproduced in any manner without written permission from the authors and publisher.

Published 2014

Cover and book design by Jennifer Miles

Printed in the United States of America

Every effort has been made to obtain permissions for pieces quoted in this work, which can be found on page 151. If any required acknowledgments have been omitted, or any rights overlooked, it is unintentional. Please notify the publisher of any omission.

Library of Congress Cataloging-in-Publication Data
Ram Dass.
  Polishing the mirror : how to live from your spiritual heart /
  Ram Dass, with Rameshwar Das ; conceived by Janaki Sandy Gaal.
     pages cm
  ISBN 978-1-60407-967-8
  1. Spiritual life. I. Das, Rameshwar. II. Title.
  BL624.R355 2013
  204'.4--dc23
                              2013005622

Ebook ISBN 978-1-62203-167-2

Enhanced ebook ISBN 978-1-62203-137-5

10 9 8 7 6 5 4 3 2 1

Dedicated to Neem Karoli Baba

*This book is a pale reflection of your light,
the flicker of a candle compared to the sun.*

Taking the pollen-like dust of my Guru's lotus feet
  to polish the mirror of my heart,
I can now sing the pure splendor of Sri Rām, the best of Raghus,
  which bestows the four fruits of life.

I don't know anything, so I remember you, Son of the Wind;
  grant me strength, intelligence, and wisdom,
  and remove my impurities and sorrows.

INVOCATION TO "HANUMAN CHALISA," TRANSLATION BY
KRISHNA DAS, FROM *FLOW OF GRACE*

Contents

Fast Foreword

THE YEAR RAM DASS'S *Be Here Now* was first published, 1971, was a turbulent time. The Vietnam War was provoking a backlash of protests. Ebullient waves from psychedelic drugs, acid rock, newfound sexual freedom, feminism, environmentalism, and back-to-the-land hippie communes were creating tectonic shifts in the existential landscape. The psychedelic expansion of consciousness began crossbreeding with Buddhism, Hinduism, and New Age spirituality to offer glimmers of internal liberation.

Idealistic visions were soon tempered by experience. There were good trips and bad trips. Deaths of students at Kent State and of rock 'n' roll heroes Jimi Hendrix, Janis Joplin, and Jim Morrison were sobering shocks. Woodstock was over. The big party woke up the morning after, smelling the coffee and needing to get on with it, laying the foundations for real change.

Richard Alpert had been Timothy Leary's professorial colleague and psychedelic sidekick at Harvard, which fired them both in 1963. After Harvard, they ran a counterculture exploratorium at Millbrook in upstate New York. In 1966, Alpert, the consummate psychedelic psychologist, went to India. He returned as Ram Dass, a Western yogi, and soon became a Johnny Appleseed of Eastern spirituality throughout the West.

After a second sojourn in India, from 1970 to 1972, Ram Dass again went on the road, lecturing tirelessly for two and a half decades. Over and over, he conveyed, with humor and stories and quotes, a shift from the Western achievement model of "making it happen" and "just doing it" to quieting the mind and being in the moment, being present and attentive and loving—just *being*. Going radically beyond his previous experiences, he described and manifested in himself a different state of being, transmitted from his guru in India. Some spiritual seeds sprouted. Thousands of people got the message and changed their lives in response.

The publication of his handcrafted manual of transcendence, *Be Here Now*, interjected a new note into the cacophonous cultural conversation of the '70s. Produced at a commune of graphic artists in the mountains of northern New Mexico and printed on brown wrapping paper, it was more graphic novel and artwork than text. When *Be Here Now* came out as a book, it was a powerful statement of this new way of being. Suddenly, out in the mainstream publishing world, there was this hand-hewn, counter-cultural owner's manual for consciousness.

It caught on. People passed it around to their friends, and it became a New Age bible. The message of *Be Here Now* was like a pebble dropped into the cultural pool of consciousness, and it continues to ripple out in contemporary lingo, yoga culture, in names of radio shows like NPR's *Here and Now,* in a stream of New Age literature flowing all over the spiritual map.

Be Here Now was not just a media phenomenon but part of a cultural shift in consciousness. More people now identify with eclectic nondenominational spirituality. Aging baby boomers are dealing more openly with life and death. Yoga has gone from being an exotic Eastern import to a transnational subculture. In the Internet age, being here now transcends time and space; we dwell entwined in a virtual moment. As we journey together through space on blue-marble earth, planetary awareness grows and separations dissolve. As Ram Dass would say, "*Them* is becoming *us.*"

For millions of us, *Be Here Now* opened doors to our deeper selves, clarifying and calming the tumult of insight and upheaval and helping many of us take the first step on the pilgrimage into our own heart. Since the '60s, the winding way of inner exploration has led us around many bends and up some blind alleys. The inner vision continues to pull, and we continue to follow.

Be Here Now shifted our point of view from whatever we thought was going on to seeing life as a spiritual journey. A section of it, the "Cookbook for a Spiritual Life," gave practical recipes for spiritual practice and yoga for Westerners. The simple message was, "Now that you've seen the light, this is how to live in it." That cookbook is still an essential resource, and the perennial imperative of the book's cryptic title remains: just be completely present in the moment. Just *be*.

The process of clearing our mind-fields of clutter and attachment in order to just be here now is complex and daunting. It's a multilevel game. As soon as you focus on one part of the jigsaw puzzle of your consciousness, something else that's even harder to deal with invariably grabs your attention. As Ram Dass says, "The mind is a wonderful servant, but a terrible master."

In keeping with these many levels of mind and emotion, the image of polishing the mirror is a multidimensional metaphor. Consciousness itself is a hall of mirrors. The key quality of the human soul is the ability to reflect on its own existence. Self-reflection, introspection, self-inquiry—whatever we call it—takes us through many layers of the onion of our inner being, from our most mundane, recursive thoughts to exalted states of pure awareness and unconditional love, of oneness or God-consciousness.

This internal reflection can also be seen as a process of witnessing, or simply observing our own actions, thoughts, and emotions with an attitude of tolerance and love. Witnessing helps us to detach from the external phenomena and sensory experiences, as well as from our mental narratives, our personal story lines that so thoroughly occupy our attention.

Witnessing subtly shifts how we identify ourselves. We shift from being the protagonist of our personal narrative, captivated by our thoughts and experiences, to seeing those thoughts and experiences as phenomena reflected in the calm mirror of our inner being. From being the star of our own show, we become an affectionate observer of the play.

Alongside this shift in the locus of our inner identity there is a process of external reflection, as we see our inner being reflected and projected onto every experience of the outer world. With patient spiritual practice, we can bring our external experience into ever-closer alignment with our inner being. This is yoga—not just yoga of the body, but also yoga of the mind (*jnana* yoga), yoga of the heart (*bhakti* yoga), and the yoga of selfless action (*karma* yoga).

As the veils of illusion begin to become more transparent, as we recognize the limitation of identifying solely with thoughts and experiences, with so-called objective reality, we begin to reflect a purer state of being. Removing the dust of impurities and attachments from the mirror of our heart-mind allows the light of the spirit to be reflected. As the layers become more transparent, the light shines through us, and we begin to dwell in a less content-laden, ever-clearer state of awareness. Awareness in the heart flowers into love, compassion, and wisdom.

Polishing the mirror, this process of reflecting on ourselves by witnessing and by bringing our external life into harmony with our true being, resolves when we identify fully with our soul, and these layers of being merge in our spiritual heart. Perhaps then there is a further stage when we cease to experience ourselves as separate beings, when the paradoxical relationship of subject and object merges in oneness. That last step requires something we can only call "grace."

Having a guide or guru for this process of self-reflection can provide us with the crucial feedback we need to stay focused and to keep us from being distracted not only by our own mental detours, but also by astral and other subtle planes. A true guru reflects our innermost being, our true Self, because he or she lives in that place. The guru's loving awareness of our journey, at every level, is an ever-present homing beacon on the path.

This book of Ram Dass's teachings is a toolkit to quiet the mind, open the heart, and enter into oneness. These teachings offer practical ways to be here now. Think of this book as a travel guide for the path to nowhere (*now-here*), a how-to guide for finding that precious sense of inner peace and spiritual reunion.

The methods are simple. The path is subtle. We are so close—just a thought away!

Only you can know for yourself if polishing the mirror is working. You'll know if you become quieter inside, more loving and compassionate, more peaceful and present, more content with your life.

As with any kind of inner work, there are endless opportunities for self-deception. The ego effortlessly morphs into a new, spiritual ego: "Wow, I'm getting really spiritual!" Ram Dass, with his humor and his honesty about his own path and its pitfalls, is a good model. May we treat ourselves with a degree of compassion and patience equal to his, and not take ourselves too seriously. There is, after all, nothing to be accomplished. We are just allowing ourselves to *be*.

IN LOVE,
RAMESHWAR DAS

Introduction

Being Here Now

BEING HERE NOW sounds simple, but these three words contain inner work for a lifetime. To live in the here and now is to have no regrets about the past, no worries or expectations for the future. To be fully present in each moment of existence is to live in total contentment, in peace and love. To enter into this presence is to reside in a different state of *being,* in a timeless moment, in the eternal present.

Once you touch this state of pure *being,* you can never completely forget it. You begin to see how your thoughts keep carrying you away from being in the moment. But *being* is always *here,* never more than a thought away. There's nothing to do, nothing to think about. Just *be—here and now.*

When our thinking mind subsides, what we might call our heart-mind takes over, and we can begin to live in love. Love is opening to merge with another being, whether with another person or with God (in the end they're the same). Love is the doorway to oneness with all things, to being in harmony with the entire universe. This return to oneness, to a simplicity of just *being,* of unconditional love, is what we all long for. This unified state is the real yoga, or union.

Perhaps this book will provide a new perspective from which to view your life. I hope you find living from this perspective a more meaningful and transcendent way of being in the world. To be fully present with ourselves and other beings is to focus on what is truly important in life, and by doing so, we become more conscious and loving.

PRACTICE MAKES PERFECT

Perhaps you are already an evolved soul who is separated from the One only by the most gossamer of veils, and your enlightenment will be nearly instantaneous. Or maybe you are a more tentative seeker whose mind pulls you this way and that, and you need more constant reminding of where your true Self lies. Whatever your karmic situation is, may this primer of consciousness be a useful road map to help guide you home. Home is where the heart *is*.

For most of us, it is helpful to set aside some time in each day to devote to spiritual practice, which means scheduling time in our already busy lives. The path of the heart is not hard or easy, but it takes time and intention. Traditionally the best times are early morning, while the world is still quiet, and during the evening, at the close of the day's activities.

Consider this your time to explore your own inner being, to find more of the meaning of your life. Spiritual practice offers us a chance to come back to the innate compassionate quality of our heart and to our intuitive wisdom. Like shopping for a new set of spiritual clothes, try on these practices of self-reflection, opening the spiritual heart, or selfless service, and see what fits. Then take a look in your mirror and see who you are now and what works for you.

Each of us has our own path to follow, our own karma. You have to honor your own unique path. You can't imitate someone else's trip. Listen to your heart to hear what you yourself need, take what you can use from these practices, and leave the rest.

THE ROAD HOME

In 1961, I was thirty and at the height of my academic career. I had a PhD from Stanford University, and I was a professor of social relations at Harvard. I had arrived at a pinnacle of life as I thought it should be, professionally, socially, and economically. But inside there remained an emptiness—a feeling that, with all I had, something was still missing. Here I was at Harvard, the mecca of the intellect. But when I looked into the eyes of my peers, wondering "Do you *know*?" I saw in their eyes that what I was looking for was nowhere to be found.

In a social or family setting, people looked up to me and hung on my every word because I was a Harvard professor, and they clearly assumed that I *knew*. But to me, the nature of life remained a mystery. I had a lot of knowledge, but I lacked wisdom. In this state of discontent, I filled my life with all the things I thought I wanted and that were supposed to be culturally fulfilling. I ate and drank too much. I collected material possessions and status symbols: I had a Triumph motorcycle and a Cessna airplane. I played the cello. I was sexually active. But these outer pleasures weren't giving me the answers I longed for. Deep inside, I had no real sense of satisfaction or contentment.

Another psychologist, Timothy Leary, moved into the office down the hall from me. Meeting Tim was a major turning point in my life. We became drinking buddies. I soon discovered that he had a brilliant mind—brilliant in a way that was different, more open to looking at the world in new ways.

One semester Timothy returned from the mountains of Mexico, where he had taken psychedelic mushrooms called *teonanácatl,* or "flesh of the gods." He said he had learned more from that experience than from all his training in psychology. I was intrigued. In March of 1961, I took psilocybin, a synthetic version of the magic mushrooms, and everything changed for me. I felt that psilocybin introduced me to my soul, which was independent of body and social identity. That experience expanded my consciousness and changed my view of reality.

Our explorations in psychedelics and subsequent dismissal from Harvard created a stir on local and national news and brought us a lot of notoriety. By that point there was a part of me that really didn't care about degrees and peer reviews, because the worlds I was exploring were far more interesting than academia. Psychedelics allowed me to cut through my traditional upbringing and tap into realms of mind and spirit that would not have been available by other means. When I got high, I felt like this was who I knew myself to be—a deep being, at peace, in love, and free.

I continued using psychedelics for five or six years, trying to stay in that place of enlightenment, that place of being love. I would get high and come down, get high and come down, touching that state of being love but unable to stay there. I wanted to be free, not high. Ultimately I realized this method wasn't working for me, and I began to sink into a deep despair.

In retrospect, while psilocybin, as well as LSD, was critical to my own awakening, psychedelics are not necessary to the process of coming into your Self. They can show you a possibility, but once you've seen the possibility, to keep revisiting it again and again isn't necessarily transformative. As Alan Watts used to say, "Once you've gotten the message, hang up the phone." Finally you have to live in the world and keep transforming within.

Aldous Huxley had given us a copy of *The Tibetan Book of the Dead,* and I realized that the East already had maps of these inner states that we were exploring intuitively and without reference points. So in 1966, I went to India in search of someone who knew about these spiritual planes of consciousness. For the first three months, I traveled with a friend who had a Land Rover shipped to Teheran and invited me to join him. We traveled through Afghanistan, Pakistan, India, and Nepal amidst a haze of hashish. But it was just another trip—more of the same, getting high and coming down—more of my own reality, leading to more despair.

Then one day in Kathmandu, Nepal, at a hippie restaurant called the Blue Tibetan, a strikingly tall Westerner with long blonde hair and a beard walked in. He was wearing Indian clothes, and he came over to our table and joined us. It turned out that Bhagavan Das, a twenty-three-year-old surfer from Laguna Beach, had been living in India for several years. After a short time with him, I knew he *knew* about India. I decided to travel with him to see what I could learn.

As we were traveling through Nepal and India, I would attempt to tell my usual charming stories or ask questions about where we were going. Bhagavan Das would say, "Don't think about the past; just be here now," or "Don't think about the future; just be here now." Although he was compassionate, he didn't involve himself in dealing with my emotions. There was nothing much to discuss. After several months of blisters on my feet, bouts of dysentery, and lessons in hatha yoga, Bhagavan Das said he had to go see his guru in the Himalaya foothills about his visa. He wanted to drive there in the Land Rover, which had been left in the care of an Indian sculptor with instructions to give it to me if I wanted it. So I went with Bhagavan Das.

On our way up to the hills, we stopped overnight, and I went outside to go to the toilet. Under the star-filled Indian sky, I thought about my mother, who had died the previous year of cancer of the spleen. As I was thinking about her, I experienced a powerful feeling of her presence. I didn't tell anyone about it. The Freudian psychologist in me thought, "There you go, thinking about your mother while you're on the toilet."

THE GURU, REMOVER OF DARKNESS

As we were driving up into the hills, I could tell something was going on with Bhagavan Das. Tears were streaming down his face, and he was singing holy songs at the top of his lungs. I sat in the corner of the seat, sulking. I thought of myself as a Buddhist, and I didn't want to see a Hindu guru.

We arrived at a small temple by the side of the road, and Bhagavan Das asked someone where the guru was. They said Maharaj-ji was up on the hill. Bhagavan Das went running up the hill, leaving me sitting there. Everybody was looking at me expectantly. I didn't know what to do. I didn't want to be there. I didn't want to see any guru. But finally, compelled by the social situation, not by my own choice, I went after him. I was stumbling uphill behind this giant who was running in big leaps and crying.

As we climbed the hill, we came around to a beautiful little field out of sight of the road and overlooking a valley. In the middle of the field was a little old man under a tree, sitting on a wooden bed with a blanket around him. Ten or fifteen Indians wearing white were sitting around him on the grass. With the clouds in the background, it was a beautiful tableau. I was too uptight to appreciate it. I thought it was some kind of cult.

Bhagavan Das ran up and prostrated himself in *danda pranam,* lying face down on the ground with his hands touching this old man's toes. Bhagavan Das was still crying, and the man was patting his head. I didn't know what to do. I thought this was lunacy. I was standing off to the side saying to myself, "Well, I've come here, but I'm not going to touch anybody's feet." I didn't know what this was all about. I was totally paranoid.

The old man was patting Bhagavan Das's head, and then he looked up at me. He pulled Bhagavan Das's head up and said to him in Hindi, "Have you got a picture of me?" Through his tears, Bhagavan Das said yes. Maharaj-ji said, "Give it to him."

I thought, "Gee, that's really nice, this little old man is going to give me a picture of himself. Wow." It was the first ego boost I had gotten all day, and I really needed it.

Maharaj-ji looked at me and said something that was translated as, "You came in a big car?" He was smiling.

That was the one topic I didn't want to talk about. We had borrowed the Land Rover from my friend. I felt responsible for it.

Still smiling, Maharaj-ji said, "Will you give it to me?"

I started to say it wasn't my car, but Bhagavan Das jumped up and said, "Maharaj-ji, if you want it, it's yours."

I sputtered, "You can't give him that car! That's not our car to give away."

Maharaj-ji looked up at me and said, "Do you make much money in America?"

I figured he thought all Americans were rich. I said, "Yeah, I made a lot of money in America, at one time."

"How much did you make?"

"Well, one year I made $25,000."

They all calculated that in rupees, and it was a sizable amount of money. Maharaj-ji said, "Will you buy a car like that for me?"

At that moment, I thought that I had never been hustled so fast in my life. I grew up around Jewish charities. We were good at shaking the tree, but never this good. I mean, I hadn't really even met this guy and already he'd asked me for a $7,000 car. I said, "Well, maybe."

This whole time he was smiling at me. My head was going around in circles. Everyone else was laughing because they knew he was putting me on, but I didn't know that.

He said we should go and take *prasad,* "blessed food." We were taken down to the little temple and treated royally and given beautiful food and a place to rest. This was way up in the mountains—no telephones, no lights, nothing.

After a while, we were brought back to Maharaj-ji. He said to me, "Come, sit." He looked at me and he said, "You were out under the stars last night."

"Yeah."

He said, "You were thinking about your mother."

"Mm . . . hmm. Yeah."

"She died last year?"

"Yeah."

"She got very big in the stomach before she died."

"That's right."

"Spleen. She died of spleen." He said "spleen" in English. When he said "spleen," he looked directly at me.

At that moment, two things happened simultaneously.

First, my rational mind, like a computer out of control, tried desperately to figure out how he could have known that. I went through every super-CIA paranoid scenario possible, like, "They brought me here, and this is part of the mind-screw thing. Or he's got this dossier on me. Wow, they're pretty good! But how could he know that? I didn't tell anyone, not even Bhagavan Das . . . ," and so on. But no matter how grandiose I got, my mind just couldn't handle this one. It wasn't in the instruction manual. It was beyond even my paranoid fantasies, and some of them were pretty imaginative.

Until then, I had an intellectual position on anything psychic or supernatural that happened. If I heard about it secondhand, I would say, as any good Harvard scientist would, "Well, that *is* interesting. We certainly must keep an open mind about these things. There's some interesting research being done in this field. We'll look into it."

Or if I were high on LSD, I as the observer would say, "Well, how do I know I'm not just creating this whole thing out of whole cloth anyway?" But I wasn't under any chemical influence, and this old man had just said "spleen." In English. How did he know that?

My mind went faster and faster, trying to figure out how Maharaj-ji could know this. Finally, like a cartoon computer with an insoluble problem, the bell rang and the red light went on and the machine stopped. My rational mind gave up. It just went *pouf!*

Second, at that same moment, there was a violent wrenching, a very painful pull in my chest, and I started to cry. Later I realized it was my fourth chakra, the heart center, opening. I looked up at Maharaj-ji, and he was looking back at me with total love. I realized he knew everything about me, even the things I was most ashamed of, and yet he wasn't judging me. He was just loving me with pure unconditional love.

I cried and I cried and I cried and I cried. I wasn't sad and I wasn't happy. The closest I can say is that I was crying because I was home. I had carried my big load up the hill, and now it was all done. The journey was over, and I had finished my search.

All that paranoia washed out of me, and everything else too. I was left with just a feeling of fantastic love and peace. I was in the living presence of Maharaj-ji's unconditional love. I had never been loved so completely. From that moment on, all I wanted was to touch Maharaj-ji's feet.

Later Maharaj-ji gave me a spiritual name, Ram Dass, which means "servant of God" ("Rām" is one of the Hindu incarnations of God, "Dass" means *servant*). He also sent Hari Dass Baba to me as a teacher to instruct me in yoga and renunciation for the next five months.

NOWHERE TO GO

During the months I was in yogi training at Maharaj-ji's little temple in the hills, I got really high. It felt like light was pouring out of my head.

At one point I had to go to Delhi to get my visa renewed. I went as a yogi. I had long hair and a long beard and *māla* (prayer beads), and I was wearing white. As I was walking barefoot through Connaught Circus, in the center of New Delhi, I felt the *shakti,* the spiritual energy, everywhere. I loved it. My newly spiritual ego was along for the ride too.

I put in my visa application and collected the mail from American Express. Then I went to a pure vegetarian restaurant for lunch. I was hungry, but I was maintaining my yogic purity. In India they treat holy people with great respect, but if you're a white holy man from the West, that's really very unusual. So I was doubly holy, and they were very respectful. They watched me eat. I had the vegetarian special, and I ate very consciously and yogically.

At the end they served a dessert that had two little English biscuits in it. I knew those weren't yogi food. You know, when you're pure, you can smell which food is pure and which is impure. But there is always a very oral Jewish boy in me too, and he *wanted* those cookies. So while I looked holy, I carefully edged the dish over and pushed the cookies into my bag. I looked as if I was thinking of something holy. I ate the biscuits in the alley outside the restaurant.

Then I went back up to the mountains, an eight-hour bus ride, and as I entered the temple, I went to touch Maharaj-ji's feet. I looked up at him, and he said, "How did you like the biscuits?"

SIMPLE TRUTH

I kept hoping to get esoteric teachings from Maharaj-ji, but when I asked, "How can I become enlightened?" he said things like, "Love everybody, serve everybody, and remember God," or "Feed people." When I asked, "How can I know God?" Maharaj-ji said, "The best form to worship God is in all forms. God is in everything." These simple teachings, to love, serve, and remember, became the guideposts for my life.

Maharaj-ji read people's thoughts, but beyond that, he knew their hearts. That blew my mind. In my own case, he opened my heart because I saw that he knew everything there was to know about me, even my darkest and most shameful faults, and he still loved me unconditionally. From that moment, all I wanted was to share that love.

Although he knew I would have liked to stay with him forever, in early spring of 1967, Maharaj-ji told me it was time for me to return to America.

He said not to tell anyone about him. I didn't feel ready, and I told him I didn't feel pure enough. He had me turn around and around, and he looked me up and down intently. Looking into my eyes, he said, "I don't see any impurities."

Before I left India, I was told that Maharaj-ji had given his *ashirvad,* his blessing, for my book. I replied, "What's an *ashirvad?* And what book?" I didn't start out planning to write the book that became *Be Here Now. Be Here Now* is Maharaj-ji's book.

As I sat in the Delhi airport, waiting to leave India, a group of American soldiers kept staring at me. I had long hair, a full beard, and was wearing a long white Indian robe that looked like a dress. One of the soldiers approached me and said, "What are you, some kind of yogurt?" When I got off the plane in Boston, my father, George, picked me up at the airport. He took one look at me and said, "Quick, get in the car before someone sees you." I thought, "This is going to be an interesting trip."

Forty years and one near-fatal stroke later, it is still quite a journey. Being here now is even more relevant for me. Being in the moment, at ease with whatever comes one's way, becomes contentment. This practice allows me to be present to love and serve others and to express unconditional love in the world. When you are fully in the moment, this moment is all there is. It feels like time slows down. When your mind is quiet, you enter into the flow of love, and you just flow from one moment to the next as naturally as breathing.

Whatever arises, I embrace it with love in the moment. This is my practice of polishing the mirror to reflect Maharaj-ji's love. In this moment there is just awareness and love. If someone asks me how to get into their heart, I give them this practice: I Am Loving Awareness.

In India when people meet and part they say, "Namasté," which means:

I honor the place in you
Where the entire universe resides.
I honor the place in you
Of love, of light, of truth, of peace.

I honor the place in you
Where if you are in that place in you and
I am in that place in me,
There is only one of us.

Namasté.

RAM DASS
MAUI
AUGUST 2013

Chapter 1

Polishing the Mirror

MIND FIELDS

The essence of yoga is union or becoming one with the universe. The conceptual heart of yoga, Patanjali's yoga sutras, begins with *"Yoga citta vritti nirodha,"* which means "unified consciousness comes with cessation of thoughts." Quieting the mind allows the natural depth of the spirit to manifest.

Meditation, the practice of quieting and concentrating and purifying the mind, aligning it with the spirit, is a foundation of yoga. Although it can start from the thinking mind and you can get into it through thought, meditation goes beyond the thinking mind. Meditation stems from the truth that who you really *are* is more than who you *think* you are.

The more you desire to know who you truly are and why you are here on earth, the more you are drawn to that truth. As you are pulled inward, you begin to leave behind the kinds of clinging and attachment that keep distorting and narrowing your vision.

Your mind can take you into the spirit, but it can also keep you deeply attached to your ego, to who you think you are. Western culture glorifies the mind, but there are other ways of knowing, and the thinking mind is only part of our being. The reality of oneness is greater than what is available to you through your senses and your thoughts.

Attachment to the melodrama of your ego is what keeps you from being here now. This model of who you think you are and how you think the world is constantly brings you down into separateness. These are habits of mind. Because of the nature of these attachments, you can see only what you can see, which from the ego's standpoint is a world of subject and objects, me and the material world.

A more skillful use of the intellect is contemplation. It is also a form of *jnana* (pronounced "gyān") yoga, the path of knowledge and wisdom. In this yoga of the mind, you use the mind to reflect on itself. For example, each morning, take out a holy book and work with a thought. Don't read many pages; just take one thought and sit with it for ten or fifteen minutes. Think about it throughout your day.

If we reflect on the qualities of Christ's love, or of equanimity, kindness, or compassion, we begin to take on those qualities. Sri Ramakrishna said, "If you meditate on your ideal, you will acquire its nature. If you think of God day and night, you will acquire the nature of God."

YOU CAN'T KNOW IT; YOU CAN ONLY BE IT

If you're reading this, you already recognize you're on a spiritual journey. You also may understand that, from within the illusion of our separateness, what we perceive is relative reality, what in India is referred to as *māya,* the projected illusion of subject and objects. All around you there are various levels of relative reality. In exploring the mind, it is helpful to examine those relative realities.

Many people are so totally involved in their lives that the spiritual element is irrelevant to them. They have no sense that behind their apparent reality there is another equally true reality, a spiritual dimension.

When you begin to awaken to your predicament—that you are trapped in illusion—you begin to see through the dreamlike quality of the veils of illusion. Everything you thought was real you now see as *māya* (illusion).

Motivations and desires affect our perceptions. We don't necessarily see things as *they* are. We see them as *we* are. Our desire system creates our perceptual universe. In that sense, you can say our reality is a projection of how we identify ourselves. Hari Dass, my yoga teacher at the ashram in India, once wrote on his chalkboard, "If a pickpocket meets a saint, all he sees are his pockets." In *The Lazy Man's Guide to Enlightenment,* Thaddeus Golas says, "You never have to change what you see, only the way you see it."

Gurdjieff, a great spiritual teacher who taught in Europe and America in the early decades of the twentieth century, noted that if you think you're free and you don't know you are in prison, you can't escape. Gurdjieff saw us as being in a prison of our own habits of mind. Unless we understand how we are conditioned by our desires, we remain stuck in the illusory reality they create, like a television program with a subliminal message that you are your desire repeating over and over.

BEYOND THOUGHT

In the West we get rewarded for rational knowledge and learning. But only when you see that the assumptions you've been working under are not valid, when you despair of getting there through your rational mind, does the possibility of truly changing your mind arise. Albert Einstein said, "A new type of thinking is essential if mankind is to survive and move toward higher levels." He also said, "The mind can proceed only so far upon what it knows and can prove. There comes a point where the mind takes a leap—call it intuition or what you will—and comes out upon a higher plane of knowledge, but can never prove how it got there. All great discoveries have involved such a leap."

In the Vedic lore of India, the ancient sages say there are three ways to acquire spiritual knowledge:

- First and most direct is through your own experience.
- Second, you hear about it from somebody you know who knows, and they tell you.
- Third is to study or learn from books like this with your logical mind.

What about other ways of knowing or experiencing life, ways that resonate with an inner validity and that feel intuitively right? Einstein said, "I didn't arrive at my understanding of the fundamental laws of the universe through my rational mind." He got there through intuition. Intuition is something we really don't understand, though we use it all the time. We say someone knew something intuitively. They have entered into a subjective rather than objective way of knowing. In fact, there are ways of knowing other than through the senses and through the thinking mind.

In 1906, William James wrote in *The Varieties of Religious Experience:*

> Our normal waking consciousness . . . is but one special type of
> consciousness, whilst all about it, parted from it by the filmiest of
> screens, there lie potential forms of consciousness entirely different.
> We may go through life without suspecting their existence; but
> apply the requisite stimulus, and at a touch they are there in all their
> completeness, definite types of mentality which probably somewhere
> have their field of application. . . . No account of the universe in its
> totality can be final which leaves these other forms of consciousness
> quite disregarded. How to regard them is the question. . . . They
> may determine attitudes though they cannot furnish formulas, and
> open a region though they fail to give a map. At any rate, they forbid
> a premature closing of our accounts with reality.

People first awaken to a spiritual dimension in their lives in an incredible variety of ways. Some people seem to open up to it through traumatic experiences, as people describe when they've come near death or at another moment when they touch something much deeper than the usual way they thought about things. Other people awaken through meditation or through religious experiences. Others arrive at it through sex or through drugs.

I remember lecturing in a hall once, back in the early '70s. Most of my audience at that time was young, and they tended to wear white and smile a lot and wear flowers. I wore my māla and had a long beard. In the front row there was a woman of about seventy, who had on a hat with little fake cherries and strawberries and things like that on it. She was wearing black oxfords and a print dress, and she had a black patent leather bag. I looked at her, and I couldn't figure out what she was doing in the audience. She looked so dissimilar to all the rest.

These talks were like a gathering of an explorers club, where we would come together and just share our experiences. I started to describe some of my experiences, some of which were pretty far out. I looked at her, and she was nodding with understanding. I couldn't believe that she could understand what I was talking about. I was describing experiences that I had using psychedelic chemicals, experiences that involved other planes of consciousness. I'd look over at her, and there she was, nodding away. I began to think maybe she had a problem with her neck and maybe it had nothing whatsoever to do with what I was saying. I kept watching and getting more and more fascinated and getting more and more outrageous, and she kept nodding and nodding.

At the end of the lecture, I just kind of smiled at her so intensely that she just had to come up and speak to me. She came up and said, "Thank you so much. That makes perfect sense. That's just the way I understand the universe to be."

And I said, "How do you know? I mean, what have you done in your life that brought you into those kinds of experiences?"

She leaned forward very conspiratorially, and she said, "I crochet."

And at that moment, I realized that people arrive at spiritual understanding through a much wider spectrum of experience than I ever anticipated.

Part of the process of awakening is recognizing that the realities we thought were absolute are only relative. All you have to do is shift from one reality to another once, and your attachment to what you thought was real starts to collapse. Once the seed of awakening sprouts in you, there's no choice—there's no turning back.

Actually, we all know that reality is relative; we have known it since childhood: "Row, row, row your boat, gently down the stream. Merrily, merrily, merrily, merrily, life is but a dream." Life *is* a dream.

LOSE YOUR MIND TO GAIN YOUR SOUL

One reason to practice purification is to cool out, so we're not creating so much heavy karma for ourselves. We are constantly preoccupied with the creations of our minds. Einstein again: "The true value of a human being can be found in the degree to which he has attained liberation from the self." What we strive to be liberated from are our habitual thought patterns about ourselves and the pull of our sensory experiences. Lightening up in these areas allows us to refocus on centering and calming the mind with meditation, mantra, or the practices of bhakti yoga. As these practices deepen, the higher wisdom comes.

Taming the mind is fraught with paradoxes. You have to give it all up to have it all. Turn off your mind. There is a place in you beyond thought that already knows—trust in that. Jesus tells us that unless we become like little children, we cannot enter the kingdom of heaven. That child mind, sometimes called beginner's mind in Zen, is the innocence of pure being, of unconditional love.

If we are to live in that state of pure being, something within us must die. It's like when a caterpillar transforms into a butterfly. The caterpillar does not become a flying caterpillar; it morphs into a butterfly.

This is the pathless path. Where the journey leads is to the deepest truth in you. It is really just returning to where you were initially before you got lost. Shedding the layers of the mind is like taking layers off of an onion. You peel them all away until you come to your essence. The spiritual journey is not about acquiring something outside yourself. Rather, you are penetrating the layers and veils to return to the deepest truth of your own being.

What you seek is already within you. This reality is subjective, not the outer objective reality. You may experience it as focused in the center of your chest. It can be called the soul, or in Hinduism the *Atmān,* or in Buddhism the pure Buddha-Mind. Jesus Christ said, "The kingdom of God is within you." This is the space of full awareness that is in harmony with the universe; this is wisdom itself. The full spirit of God is inside each of us. When you want to approach God, go inward.

ENLIGHTENING UP

Offering up or cleaning up the ego stuff that distracts you from the spirit is called purification. Purification is an act of letting go that is done out of discriminative awareness—that is, you understand that you are a soul passing through a life in which the entire drama is a script for your awakening and that you are more than just the drama. You are a spiritual being having a human experience. Your life experience is a vehicle for coming to God, for becoming conscious, for becoming liberated. Ultimately that's what you are doing here. This awareness helps you discriminate between thoughts, feelings, and actions that bring you closer to God, to your own freedom, and those that take you away from it.

Instead of filling your mind with the daily news, fill it with stuff that helps you become more conscious, that liberates you. As you become more aware of what gets you to God and what doesn't, you will naturally let go of what doesn't. That's purification. You do it to get to God, not for the sake of being pure.

So how do you become conscious of all these unconscious influences? Go within to your spiritual heart, your *hridayām, and watch the drama that is your entire life. When you quiet your mind enough to transcend your ego, you can begin to hear how it all is.* Then you watch with unbearable compassion for yourself and all beings. Watching involves what you may call the witness consciousness, which comes from your soul plane. It is another way of polishing the mirror, to connect your thinking mind with your spiritual heart.

You observe your behavior and thoughts, enhancing your ability to live fully in the moment, to be here now. Then, when you are with a candle flame, you *are* the candle flame and the watcher. When there is a task to do, you *are* the task and the observer of the task. It's not that you do it—it's *how* you do it, where you are coming from as you act.

WATCHING THE WATCHER

The witness doesn't evaluate; it doesn't judge your actions. It merely makes note of them. It's a subtle thing, the watcher watching him- or herself watching. It's actually two planes of consciousness simultaneously, the witness and the ego. The witness is connected to the soul plane.

At first, you may be distracted and remember to witness only now and then. Later you'll notice that although you still fall asleep and lose the witness, you start to remember to witness again sooner. Just notice. You don't have to change anything. Eventually things will change naturally. After some practice, it gets more subtle, and throughout the day you remain centered in the witness, watching life's drama unfold. The witness is always here and now. It resides in each instant of living.

You ask yourself, "How do I use my every moment to get here?" The attitude is not heavy or tight, like "I've got to be careful; I might make a mistake." Relax, be light, dance through it all, trusting, quieting, flowing. Your witnessing lives in the flow of your love and the quietness of your mind. Women in Indian villages talk and gossip as they walk back from the well, but they never forget the jugs of water on their heads. The jug of water is what your journey is all about. So do what you do in your life, but don't forget the jug of water. Don't forget what it's all about.

The illusion keeps pulling you back into forgetting. Lost in your melodrama, you keep forgetting into it. Sometimes you spill the water. You will keep forgetting and remembering and forgetting and remembering. And every now and then, *you remember.* Keep your eye on the mark.

BREATHING IN,
BREATHING OUT

Eventually the balance shifts. You allow your life to become simpler and more harmonious. Less and less you grab at this and push away that. You listen to hear how it is rather than imposing a structure. Imposing structures doesn't set you free. Your romantic attachment to your own story line and how it comes out fades. "Who am I becoming?" and "What will I be when I grow up?" are irrelevant when you are just *being.* All of these models just fall away. You start to sit simply, live simply, just be where you are, just be with whomever you're with when you're with them. You listen for your *dharma,* the spiritual way of living your life.

Aldous Huxley reminds us, "The body is always in time, the spirit is always timeless and the psyche is an amphibious creature compelled by the laws of man's being to associate itself to some extent with its body, but capable, if it so desires, of experiencing and being identified with its spirit."

Your whole life becomes a meditative act. It's not just sitting on your meditation pillow, your *zafu*. All of life is a big zafu, no matter whether you're driving or making love or whatever you're doing. It's all meditation. It is the practice of being here now.

When you meditate, you begin to develop the power of your mind through concentration, through one-pointedness, by following the breath or repeating a mantra. You develop the capacity to put your mind on one thought and keep it there and let everything else flow by. You don't stop your mind. You let it flow. But you bring one thought constantly to the surface. You keep coming back to one thought. "Breathing in, breathing out," or "Rising, falling." Or you use your mantra, "Rām, Rām, Rām, Rām, Rām . . ." Whether you are eating, sleeping, making love, "Rām, Rām, Rām . . ." keeps going. You spiritualize your life. You convert it all by maintaining a frame of reference that has the dual capacity of centering you and increasing the power of one-pointedness. Maharaj-ji told me, "Bring your mind to one point and wait for grace."

A GUIDED VISUAL MEDITATION

Sit straight, so your head, neck, and chest are in alignment. Start by focusing in your heart area, in the middle of your chest, where the hridayām, the spiritual heart, is located. With your mouth closed, breathe in and out of your chest, focusing on your heart as if you were breathing in and out through your heart. Breathe deeply.

Because of the purity of your seeking, many incredibly high beings are present, and with them comes the spiritual substance out of which all form derives. You can imagine that substance as a golden mist that fills the air. With every breath, don't just breathe in air; imagine you are pulling into yourself this golden substance. Fill with it; let it pour through your entire body.

Breathe in the energy of the universe, the *shakti* of the universe. Breathe in the breath of God. Let it fill your whole body. Each time you breathe out, breathe out all of the things in you that keep you from knowing your true Self; breathe out all the separateness, all the feelings of unworthiness, all the self-pity, all the attachment to your pain, whether it's physical or psychological. Breathe out anger and doubt and greed and lust and confusion. Breathe in God's breath, and breathe out all the impediments that keep you from knowing God. Let the breath be the transformation.

Now let the golden mist that has poured into your being focus in the middle of your chest; let it take form as a tiny being, the size of a thumb, sitting on a lotus flower right in the middle of your chest. Notice its equanimity, the radiance that comes from within. Use your imagination. As you look upon this being, see that it is radiating light. See the light pouring out. As you meditate upon it, experience the deep peace that is emanating from this being. Feel, as you look upon this being, that it is a being of great wisdom. It's sitting quietly, silently, perfectly poised in your heart. Feel its compassion and its love. Let yourself be filled with its love.

Now, slowly let that tiny being grow in size until it fills your body, so its head fills the space of your head, its torso, your torso, its arms, your arms, its legs, your legs. So now in the skin of your body sits this being—a being of infinite wisdom, a being of the deepest compassion, a being that is bathed in bliss, a being that is self-effulgent: a being of perfect tranquility.

Let this being begin to grow in size. Experience yourself growing until everything in the room around you is within your body. All of the sounds, all the sensory experiences are coming from inside you.

Continue to grow. Feel your vastness, your peace, your equanimity. Your head extends into the sky. Expand until your town, your environment, and all those beings within them are contained within you. Experience the human condition; see the loneliness, joy, caring, violence, paranoia, a mother's love for her child, sickness, fear of death—see it all. It is all within you. See it with compassion and with caring and, at the same moment, with equanimity. Feel the light pour through your being.

Let yourself grow still larger. Feel your vastness increase until you are sitting in the middle of this galaxy, the earth deep within your belly. All humankind is within you. Feel the turmoil and the longing. Feel the beauty. Sit in this universe, silent, peaceful, compassionate, loving. All of the creations of human beings' minds are within you; look upon them with compassion.

Continue to grow until not only this galaxy but every galaxy is within you, until everything you can conceive of is within you. All of it is inside you. You are the only One. Feel your aloneness, your silence, your peace. There are no other beings here; all planes of consciousness are within you, and all beings are within you.

You are the Ancient One. Everything that ever was, is, or will be is part of the dance of your being. You are the universe, so you have infinite wisdom; you feel all of the feelings of the universe, so you have infinite compassion. Let the boundaries of your being dissolve, and merge yourself into that which is beyond form. Sit for a moment in the formless, beyond compassion, beyond love, beyond God. Let it all be in its perfection.

Very gently, very slowly, let the boundaries of your vast being, the One, reestablish themselves. Vast, silent, all is within you. Come back from beyond the One and slowly come down in size. Come down through the universes into this universe, until your head is once again among the planets and the earth is within you. Come down again until your head is once again in the heavens and the cities are within you.

Come down in size until your head is at the top of your room. Stop here for a moment. From this place, look down into the room and find the being who you thought you were when you began this meditation. Look at that being, bringing to bear all of your love and compassion. See the journey of that being as it is living out this incarnation; see its fears, its doubts, its connections. See all the thoughts and objects it clings to that keep it from being free. See how close it is to knowing who it is. Look within that being and see the purity of its soul.

Reach down and, with your mind, very gently place your hand on the head of this being and bestow upon it your blessing that in this very life it may fully know itself. Experience simultaneously that which blesses and that which is being blessed.

Now come back down into the body you thought you were when you began. You are still flesh surrounding a being of radiance and wisdom, a being of compassion that comes from attunement with the truth, with love for all that comes from being that vast One. That love and peace are pouring out of you to all beings everywhere, like a beacon for all those who suffer.

Remember those people toward whom you have felt less than loving. Look to their souls and surround them with light, with the love and peace of this moment. Let go of the anger and the judgment.

Send the light of love and peace out to people who are ill, who are lonely, who are afraid, who have lost their way. Share your blessings, because only when you give can you continue to receive. As you journey on this spiritual path, accept the responsibility for sharing what you receive. That is part of God's harmony, of becoming an instrument for the will of God.

Let the radiant, perfect being within you again assume its diminutive form, the size of a thumb. See it again sitting on a lotus flower in your spiritual heart, in the middle of your chest, radiant with light, peaceful, immensely compassionate. This being is love. This being is wisdom. This is the inner guru. This is the being within you who always *knows*. This is the being you meet through your deeper intuition when you go beyond your mind. This is the tiny form of the entire universe that exists within you.

At any time, you need only sit and quiet your mind, and you will hear this being guiding you home. When you finish this journey, you will have disappeared into this being, surrendered, merged, and then you will know the truth that Ramana Maharshi, a great realized being from India, meant when he said that God, guru, and Self are one.

Chapter 2

Bhakti Yoga,
the Path of Devotion

"YOGA" MEANS "YOKE" or "union"—union with God. Bhakti yoga is the path of devotion, of loving God and imbibing God's love. The practitioner of bhakti, the *bhakta,* is the lover, and God is the Beloved. Bhakti uses the dualism of relationship, the deep longing of the heart, for the lover to merge with the Beloved, to become one in love. Bhakti is the path of the spiritual heart, using our human emotions to forge the connection between the human and the divine. The practices of bhakti yoga awaken this flow of love.

We may sing to the Beloved, we may pray, we may sit with a picture of a holy being, or we may just dwell in the sweetness of remembering God. Once you have set out on the river of love, all you have to do is let it carry you to the ocean. When Maharaj-ji was asked how to meditate, he said, "Meditate the way Christ meditated. . . . He lost himself in love."

Devotion complements the quieting of the mind in meditation by opening the heart. This outflowing of the heart toward the object of our devotion further polishes the mirror reflecting the spirit. This flow of loving energy amplifies other methods too, as we'll explore later.

Opening my heart made it easier for my mind to change. That's really what devotion is about—it's a way of making it very easy to turn your mind in a certain direction because the love is so seductive, because it brings so much joy. Ramakrishna said, "Bhakti, love of God, is the essence of all spiritual discipline."

The yoga of devotion starts from right here where we are, as embodied souls separate from God. When we are fully present in this moment, with a quiet mind and an open heart, we experience the flow of love from our spiritual heart. Bhakti yoga opens us to this flow of divinely inspired love.

You could say bhakti is the love play, the *līla*, between God and the soul. Bhakti yoga uses the dualistic relationship of lover and Beloved to take us into the essence of love, to become love. Love has a built-in power to carry us beyond the limitations of our separate being, our ego, to the Atmān, our higher being. Our personal emotional love gets absorbed into the all-encompassing unconditional love of the One. As Meher Baba said, "Being is dying by loving."

Of all the different yogas, all the many ways to the One, all the various routes up the mountain, bhakti is known as the easy path. With bhakti, you don't really have to *do* anything; you just relax and let go and open your heart.

It doesn't matter whether you call it love of God or of the guru or of the truth of who you are. How you think of it is really irrelevant. The emotional tidal wave of a love affair with the Divine is so intense that it carries you beyond your thinking mind. This devotion begins to permeate whatever you're doing in your life, bringing it into the divine love play. In Sanskrit that soul joy is called *sāt cit anānda*, "truth-consciousness-bliss." Or you could say, "Consciousness of Truth is bliss."

Devotion to God underlies most spiritual traditions, especially those oriented more to the emotional and ecstatic than to the intellectual. Love is more than an idea. We can't just sit down and intellectually figure out what bhakti or devotion is about. It has to do with the heart, and heart trips are experienced in a realm that's not necessarily conceptual. The harder you try to think your way through to devotion, the harder it will be. Hafiz the poet said, "O thou who are trying to learn the marvel of love from the copybook of reason, I'm very much afraid that you will never really see the point."

We can think and talk about bhakti yoga, but we *experience* it through *kirtan,* or chanting; mystical poetry; the remembrance of saints; mantras for opening the heart; or just by being together in love, in true *satsang.* The openness of love is timeless. When you are with another being in love, you are sharing your being, your presence. You are just here, together in love.

The minute I heard my first love story
I started looking for you, not knowing how blind that was.

Lovers don't finally meet somewhere.
They are in each other all along.
RUMI

Many of us are afraid to let go of our judging minds to fall into love, to be absorbed into the liquid flow of the universe. In the case of divine love, faith makes it easier to let go. In romantic relationships it's a tricky balance because relationships bring up our personal fears and vulnerabilities. Understanding the difference between emotional or romantic love and divine love is helpful in allaying those fears. Loving God is totally safe because the object of love is ultimately your true Self.

In *Cutting Through Spiritual Materialism,* the Tibetan teacher Chogyam Trungpa Rinpoche speaks of what is necessary for a spiritual transmission between two people—a relationship of openness and trust and warmth. Another expression of that relationship is from the *I Ching:* "The Master said . . . when two people are at one in their inmost hearts, they shatter even the strength of iron or of bronze. And when two people understand each other in their inmost hearts, their words are sweet and strong, like the fragrance of orchids."

HOW DO I LOVE THEE?

Gurdjieff talks about three levels of love. There's physiological, sexual, biochemical love—"let's make love." Then there is romantic love, which is personality love, loving an object. Romantic love has in it jealousy and possessiveness and all the interpersonal psychodynamics. When you say, "I fell in love with so-and-so," what you are really saying is, "So-and-so turns me on to the place in me where I *am* the ocean of love."

The third kind of love is conscious love, spiritual love. It is important to understand that there is a difference between romantic love and spiritual love. To change romantic love into an expanding, conscious love, we have to take it up another level. Conscious or spiritual love is unconditional; it's soul love. To enter into the space of conscious love you *become* love—not loving someone or something, but just *being* love.

This is not to say these levels of love are really separate or that one kind can't be contained in another, such as sexual love becoming subsumed in love of the Divine (a practice of *Tantra*, a yoga that uses external energy for internal transformation). Bhakti focuses on spiritual love, the soul's love for God.

If we can see even for a moment that loving another person *is* loving the manifestation of the spirit in them, just loving love, then they become yet another form of the Beloved, of God. This is love's truth: that love is in all of us, that we are one in love.

Rām hi kewal prema piyara
Jnani leo jo ja nani hara

Love loves only love
He who knows this can know
FROM THE *RAMAYANA* OF TULSI DAS

LOVE IS A STATE OF BEING

When I live in the place where I *am* love, I see love wherever I look. It's very far out. Imagine seeing love in everyone and everything. Love doesn't demand that you do anything about it. We're all right here in love. To the extent another being is open, when I meet them, there's a harmonic resonance with the place where they also exist as love—not that they are *loving*, but where they *are* love. Suddenly here we are in the ocean of love, which is what Christ's love is about. This love isn't possessive. We can't collect it. We can only become it.

As you grow in devotion and focus more and more on the Beloved, you tune in to a deeper place within yourself. The emotional, romantic qualities give way to a new kind of love where finally you see everyone and everything as the Beloved.

It is only when you begin to understand that love is a state of being that you can really *be* in love. If you and I are truly in love, if we both dwell in the place in ourselves that is love, we are together in love. Being in love is sharing a common state together.

Anandamayi Ma, the Indian saint whose name means "bliss-permeated mother," said to her devotees, "You all love this body so much that you often come to see me, unmindful of the long distance that many of you have to travel. Yet, it is true that this body has no relationship with any of you except the kinship of the Atmān [the universal soul] which this body enjoys equally not only with each of you but even with all trees, creepers, and foliage around, as well as with rocks, mountains and everything else."

GURU KRIPA (THE GURU'S GRACE)

When Dada Mukerjee, an old devotee of Maharaj-ji, visited the Neem Karoli Baba Ashram in Taos, New Mexico, he was surprised to find sincere devotees who had never met Maharaj-ji in the body. Dada said, "The real miracle is these devotees who never met Maharaj-ji and have the same devotion." They knew Maharaj-ji primarily through the stories in *Be Here Now* and *Miracle of Love*. Many Westerners have realized that if you invite Maharaj-ji into your heart, he will be with you.

That quality of loving, trusting openness allows you to receive the transmission from another being. It was Maharaj-ji's love and my opening to him that allowed his blessings to come through. The way bhakti works is you just love until you and the Beloved become one. As each person opens and loves, the grace comes through—it just pours into you.

Let me always feel you present,
in every atom of my life.

Let me keep surrendering my self
until I am utterly transparent.
Let my words be rooted in honesty
and my thoughts be lost in your light,
Unnamable God, my essence,
my origin, my life-blood, my home.
FROM PSALM 19, TRANSLATED BY STEPHEN MITCHELL

For me, the form of the Beloved is my guru, Maharaj-ji Neem Karoli Baba. Because the guru is so much a part of my path, I am often asked if it is necessary to have one. It depends on how you understand what a guru is. As you go deeper, you begin to understand (as the meditation at the end of the last chapter shows) that God, guru, and Self are indeed one.

So the answer comes on different levels. On one hand, it's not necessary to have an external guru, because the true guru is an internal relationship. In the higher sense of Self, you *are* the guru. On the other hand, as long as you identify yourself as a separate entity, it can be helpful to have a personal guru to keep you headed in the right direction. It depends on what you need.

In bhakti yoga the form of your Beloved can be whatever you love deeply. You can find it in God, in a guru, in a teacher, in a flower, or a pet. The Beloved is everywhere. You can find the Beloved in anyone or anything you love deeply enough that opens your heart and takes you through. Just allow that love to open you and dissolve the boundaries of your separateness, melding into one.

Listen to the messages that come through as you sit quietly, and you will find plenty of guidance. The quieter your mind gets, the more you are able to hear these inner messages and allow them to guide you.

How will you know your guru? The guru will know you. You don't have to look for the guru. The guru appears when you are ready. You'll know. There won't be any doubt. The guru is a mirror that reflects your higher Self, allows you to see that place of love and pure being in yourself. The guru may be Christ or any of a number of beings, and not necessarily on the physical plane.

Your guru will guide you, to the extent that you ask purely, through one teaching after another. Some teachings may take the form of other teachers or situations or experiences. Other teachings may come from inner experiences as you quiet inside and deepen your practice. As you begin to trust in that relationship, you will become more and more attuned to that presence and awareness. Ask your guru to guide you, and you will begin to see how each life situation is a teaching from your guru to bring you home.

In India it is understood that you do not seek the guru. Rather, it is the guru who finds you.

A guru is different from a teacher. A teacher points the way; the guru *is* the way. The guru beckons from beyond. He or she is somebody who's all finished. A teacher or teaching, on the other hand, is somebody (or something) standing next to you and pointing up the road.

Most people we call gurus are really teachers whose goose is not fully cooked. The likelihood of finding a being who is completely done is fairly slim. Most teachers are still working out their own karma; they have their own stuff still to resolve. A teacher can be someone through whom a teaching comes, though they themselves may not *be* the full truth.

From your point of view, if you're seeking truth with a pure heart, you separate the purity of a teacher's message from the stuff of their karma. That discrimination develops as you listen to the guru inside, to your Self. Then you take a teacher's truth, and you work with it and use it to take you further on your path. The rest is their karma.

Even your enemies can be teachers who wake you up to a place that you're not, that you need to bring into your awareness. They help you get free of that place and get on with it. If you see everything in the universe as a way to work on your own consciousness—even if it's showing you where you're unconscious or where you're asleep—then everyone and everything in the universe becomes your teacher and a means of awakening.

My own teachers have come in all kinds of packages. Some years ago I was invited by John and Toni Lilly to swim with their dolphins, Joe and Rosie. Everybody wanted to swim with dolphins, and I wanted to swim with dolphins too, although I wasn't quite sure why. When I got to the holding tank, it was a cold, gray day. I thought maybe this was really not for me. But other people were watching, and after all, this was Ram Dass swimming with the dolphins.

I got into the water, and these huge beings zoomed by me very close up. They were quite intimidating. I was treading water and feeling out of my natural medium. After a while, one of the dolphins, Rosie, was sort of hovering just to my left, and I reached out and touched her. I assumed that when you touch a wild creature it would be startled or irritated and swim away. But Rosie didn't swim away.

I started to stroke Rosie's back. It was amazingly soft, like silk, very porous. I stroked some more. The wild creature model of who I had thought she was had stopped working. In that model, she wouldn't have allowed me to stroke her because I was doing it with considerable pressure at that point. In that moment, my mind let go, and I started to experience ecstasy just being with Rosie. Then she dove to the bottom of the pool, but I stayed on the surface. When I didn't follow her to the bottom, she came back up to get me. When I finally let go, Rosie turned herself upright, vertical in the water, and pressed her stomach against my stomach.

I noticed everyone watching me with my stomach pressed against this dolphin's stomach, and I wondered, "Is this legal? Is it ethical?" I found myself putting my arms around her and kissing her on the mouth, saying, "Oh, Rosie!" I was going into such states of ecstasy. I realized that Rosie, as one of my teachers, was taking me out of my mind into the fullness of the moment that is part of the mystery of enlightenment.

Teachings are everywhere. Your guru is waiting for you to be ready for him or her. You don't have to rush off to India, because the guru and the teaching are always right where you are, right here, right now.

DIVINE RELATIONSHIPS

Devotion is a love affair between your soul and God. K. K. Sah, one of Maharaj-ji's closest devotees, was with Maharaj-ji since childhood. Maharaj-ji assigned him to watch over me, and he took me to live in his home in those early days in India. Here is what he writes about devotion:

Devotion is easy and natural and has no hard and fast rules on how one should meditate. By devotion one can realize the secret of love itself. On this path the aspirant sees the universe as the very expression of his Beloved.

The only thing it requires is faith—implicit faith. There is nothing to argue, it is beyond logic. It is like learning to swim: a person cannot enter the water unless he can swim, and swimming is impossible without entering the water.

There are various attitudes or feelings with which one may approach the Beloved. You might feel as though God were your child, like the feeling of Yashoda (Krishna's mother) toward her baby Krishna, or the feeling of Mary for the infant Jesus. Or you could see God as a friend. Again there is the attitude of the servant toward his Master, where you serve the Lord as Hanuman serves Lord Rama in the Ramayana. Then there is the attitude of lover, where you see your Beloved with the love of husband or wife. . . . Becoming the bride of God, like the Gopis sporting with Lord Krishna or St. Therese the Little Flower married to her Beloved Jesus. Finally there is the attitude of peaceful contemplation of the great saints and sages, the ancient yogis of India.

There are many ways to open yourself, to make yourself more receptive to this love for God. One way is through satsang, the company of Saints, contact with the living spirit of truth and love in other beings. Delighting in the stories and incidents of God in His many forms and incarnations—like the life of Christ, or Rama or Krishna—can also bring this love. Or by humbly serving at the feet of the Guru, the devotee can efface the ego in surrender to God. And constantly singing His name and His praises further centers the mind and heart on Him. For the devotee, the mere repetition of the Name of God brings His Presence. Then with firm faith, one crosses the ocean of desire in the boat of the Name.

MAHARAJ-JI

The method of the guru is called *guru kripa,* which is the particular form of bhakti yoga that focuses on the guru and on the guru's blessing or grace (kripa). Most of the time I'm just hanging out with my guru, even though he's no longer in the body. The thoughts and remembrances of him come up a thousand times a day. I may be sitting with someone, and they turn into my guru—over and over again. It's just hanging out with this incredible being of love, of consciousness, of presence. It's a way of opening myself to those qualities. It's a process of surrendering to that place of unconditional love.

The essence of a relationship with a guru or spiritual teacher is love. The guru awakens incredible love in us, then uses that love to help us out of the illusion of duality.

The relationship between the guru and the *chela* ("devotee") was beautifully described by Ramana Maharshi: "It's like an elephant waking up upon seeing a lion in a dream. Just as the appearance of the dream lion is enough to wake the elephant, so also is the glance of Grace from the Master enough to waken the devotee from the sleep of ignorance to the Knowledge of the Real." In other words, the guru, as a separate entity, exists only within the illusion of separateness, within the dream. As soon as the method of the guru has worked and it awakens you, it automatically self-destructs.

The relationship between a guru and a chela has nothing to do with the intellect whatsoever. You may think you're surrendering, but there's really no choice involved in it. There is just deep karma unfolding so that you are drawn to the guru when the moment is right.

At first all I wanted to do was be with my guru, look at his form, and touch his feet. After a while, the love grew different, no less intense but less to do with the form, until I was very fulfilled just being at a distance from him. And as time went on, it just kept growing deeper and deeper, and I didn't care if I was with his form at all anymore. As I went deeper still, it wasn't about a man in India anymore—it was the essence of *guruness.* I began to experience it in myself instead of in relation to him as an external being. The whole dynamic of the relationship was changing as I was deepening and my heart was opening and my surrender was increasing. I've said half jokingly that I worshiped his form until I realized his form was just the doorpost and I was just worshiping doorposts. As I looked through that doorway, each surrender led me further in. It was a method that took me right back into myself and beyond the form.

The guru constantly reflects back that part of us that is beyond form. That process also illuminates the dust on our own mirror, the impurities and imperfections of our individuality that keep us from becoming one, from living fully in that place of pure being and unconditional love. Sometimes, for a moment, the guru will blow it away to give us a glimpse.

I remember standing in the front yard of a humble house in a village in the hills when Maharaj-ji arrived unexpectedly. I was told to remain outside, so I had the opportunity to watch other people arriving. They seemed to appear almost out of nowhere, coming from all directions. Women were running, wiping flour from their hands on their aprons, carrying their half-dressed babies. The men had left their shops unattended. People were pulling flowers from the trees as they came, so they would have something to offer. They came with a feeling of expectation, with such joy and a reverence that could not be mistaken.

I watched newcomers arrive, some skeptical with questions. I saw their hearts gently open and this soft, flowerlike quality emerge under the tender care of the master gardener. Maharaj-ji touched each person's heart in a way special to that individual. Everyone's experience with him was different. That's why you can't explain what it was like to be with him. Everyone had their own heart connection.

How do you describe a being like Maharaj-ji? It's like trying to describe the sweetness of a fruit or the fragrance of a rose. When I was with him, there was nothing other than Maharaj-ji—it was total, effortless worship. Krishna Das remembers, "We would come up against our fears and our stuff, and then he'd just kill it with love. Maharaj-ji would just look at you and giggle, and you would forget your stuff." He was like a magnet of love attracting us all. And that love was his real teaching.

For some devotees, what stands out is the precious intimacy that comes from experiencing another being within the same space that your own being occupies, like the whisper of a lover who knows your innermost heart. When you are in the presence of unconditional love, you are in the optimum environment for your heart to open. The moment your heart opens, you are once again letting in the flow, and that flow is where you experience God. That is the experience of being with Maharaj-ji. Perhaps your experience with your Beloved is like that too.

Meher Baba, in *Life at Its Best*, said, "Devotees should keep their love for their Guru alive and aglow, by making him their constant companion in all their thoughts, words and actions, while carrying on their responsibilities, commitments and all other apparently necessary things of this world."

THE FEELING OF DEVOTION

I will set You on my breath
So You will become my life.
RUMI

Swami Muktananda, in his guru kripa *sadhana*, used to meditate intensely on his guru, Nityananda. He would visualize bringing him into his own body until he himself became Nityananda. So intoxicated did he become in his devotion to his guru that there were times when he didn't know if he was Muktananda or Nityananda.

A sense of that feeling of devotion comes from the first-century Odes of Solomon:

My heart was split, and a flower appeared;
*   and grace sprang up; and it bore fruit for my God.*
You split me, tore my heart open,
*   filled me with love.*
You poured your spirit into me;
*   I knew you as I know myself.*

. . .

My eyes are radiant with your spirit;
my nostrils fill with your fragrance.
My ears delight in your music,
and my face is covered with your dew.
Blessed are the men and women
who are planted on your earth, in your garden,
who grow as your trees and flowers grow,
who transform their darkness to light.
Their roots plunge into darkness;
their faces turn toward the light.

. . .

There is infinite space in your garden;
all men, all women are welcome here;
all they need do is enter.

HANUMAN, DEVOTED SERVANT OF RĀM

The Indian epic the *Rāmayana* is a saga of God taking physical form as a warrior prince to guide humanity and strengthen our faith. It's a story of grace. The legend is that it was first written down in Sanskrit over 2,000 years ago by the poet-sage Valmiki. A vernacular Hindi version by Tulsi Das is recited and performed in Hindu homes and temples and at annual festivals. It's like the Bible of North India. You can read the *Rāmayana* on many levels, as an actual historic event or a romantic tale of the battle between good and evil. You can also hear the characters as symbolic archetypes of sacred and secular forces, the soul and the ego, the truth of dharma and the illusion of desire, all of which vie within each of us. It is a multilevel work of living spirit that stirs our impulses toward divinity.

One of the main characters in the *Rāmayana* is the monkey god, Hanuman, who is the perfect servant and great devotee of Rām— God in the human form of a prince. Hanuman represents our simian lower nature in service of the highest Self. Hanuman says to Rām, "When I don't know who I am, I serve you. When I know who I am, you and I are one."

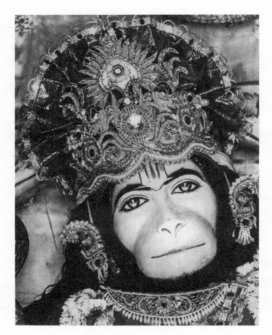

Hanuman

Rām and his wife, Sita, and his brother, Lakshman, were banished to the forest for fourteen years under extraordinary circumstances. (You will have to read the book if you want all the details.) Sita, the perfect wife, who is also the soul and the earth mother, the *shakti* or power of God, is stolen away, kidnapped by Ravana, a demon king who is the bad guy in the story. Ravana is full of ego and pride. He has ten heads, and every one of them is full of power. Rām, though he is God on Earth, is distraught because he's also a husband. (As a husband he's bereft, though as God, he's not.)

Looking for Sita, Rām enlists the help of the bears and the monkeys, who are rather human characters too. The chief monkey to help him is Hanuman. They search for Sita and finally ascertain that she has been taken by Ravana to the island of Sri Lanka (which used to be called Ceylon) off the southern coast of India.

There is an ocean between India and Sri Lanka, and when the monkeys and bears all get to the shore, they can't figure out how to get across to rescue Sita. They're discussing it among themselves, and each one has a reason why they can't jump across. Somebody has to just jump the ocean; there's no time for anything else.

Finally they turn to Hanuman, who is just sitting there kind of meekly. "Hanuman, you haven't said anything."

Now, Hanuman is under a curse because of some mischief he got into when he was a young monkey and inadvertently disturbed a yogi. Otherwise he has all the power in the universe, since he lives only to serve God. But he's cursed to have no self-consciousness of his own power (just as you or I really have no sense of our true inner power). One of his companions says, "Hanuman, you have the power to leap the ocean."

He says, "Oh, I do? Oh yes, of course, I can jump over the ocean."

At that point, he starts to grow in size from just a regular monkey into a huge, huge form. This is really just a symbol of the leap of faith that each of us has to make, to have faith in ourselves and faith in the universe, faith in the flow of things, to go beyond ourselves.

Hanuman leaps across the ocean as Rām's messenger to locate Sita and reassure her that Rām has not forgotten her. Sita, the perfect devotee of Rām, represents all devotees. Hanuman is serving God by reminding the devotee to have faith—that God cannot possibly forget us.

This is from William Buck's version of the *Rāmayana*:

In his mind Hanuman had already crossed the sea and entered the demon city. He climbed one of the Malaya hills to get firm ground under his feet. He began to fill up with power. He grew very large and heavy, and his tread pressed down on the hill and crushed the caves of the serpents. Out from the underworld came the richly dressed Nagas [the serpent gods], bruised and hissing, their hoods spread wide. In their anger they rolled on the ground with tongues flaming. They spat fire and bit the rocks in passion. Their venom cracked the hill, and gleams of red metal and stone shone from within the Earth.

Hanuman climbed higher. With smiles of amazement, the heavenly Gandharvas [the astral musicians] and their Apsarasas rose half-dressed from the hill into the sky and looked down to watch. Hanuman climbed up through their hillside parks, where Gandharva swords and bright colored robes were hung on trees, and golden wine cups and silver dishes were on the ground in fair shady gardens hiding lovers' beds of lotus petals.

Hanuman neared the summit. His feet squeezed water from the hill. Rivers tumbled down, rockslides rolled, bright fresh-broken veins of gold sparkled, tigers ran off and birds flew away. The tree spirits fled, and in their dens the wild cats yelled in a frightful chorus like the cry of the mountain himself through the voice of all his animals.

Hanuman stood on the hilltop. He held his breath and sucked in his stomach. He frisked his tail and raised it a little at the end. He bent his knees and swung back his arms, and on one finger gleamed Rama's gold ring [that he was taking to Sita]. Then without pausing to think he drew in his neck, laid back his ears and jumped.

It was grand! It was the greatest leap ever taken. The speed of Hanuman's jump pulled blossoms and flowers into the air after him and they fell like little stars on the waving treetops. The animals on the beach had never seen such a thing; they cheered Hanuman, then the air burned from his passage, and red clouds flamed over the sky and Hanuman was far out of sight of land.

That white monkey was like a comet, pushing the sky from his way and bumping clouds aside. The wind roared under his arms and was pushed down from his breast as he passed, and made the ocean pitch and roll. Sea spray rose and steamed up the Sun. Beneath Hanuman as he went, the green salt water parted, and he could see the whales and fishes like people surprised at home. The air around Hanuman became electric, and sheets of light gathered and crackled—blue, and pale melon green, and flickering orange and red.

Halfway across to Lanka, the golden mountain Mainaka lived on the ocean floor, and from under sea he saw Hanuman coming and thought he would be tired. . . .

"Rest awhile," said Mainaka. "Let me pay my ancient debt to your father, the Wind." . . .

"Forgive me, but I must not break my flight," said Hanuman.

What a glorious leap! A leap into the unknown, a leap way beyond Hanuman's capacity, a leap way beyond who he thought he was. Your own leap—your leap into life, into death, into the next moment, into freedom—comes from giving up the model of who you think you are. Who are you? Are you a straight person? Are you a clown? Have you been laughing forever? Have you been sad long enough? Is it all very heavy and important? Or is it kind of light and playful? How does this round work for you? It's all wide open this time. It's all wide open.

On Hanuman's return, after he has found Sita and leapt back across the ocean, Rām praises and embraces him in a moment of divine affection. Hanuman, ever the humble servant, responds, "Save me, save me (from the tentacles of egoism), my lord!"

Rām says, "As long as men shall speak of you, you will live on Earth. No one can equal you. Your heart is true; your arms are strong; you have the energy to do anything. You have served me faithfully and done things for me that couldn't be done."

"It's nothing," said Hanuman, "I am your friend, that's all."

Hanuman is the connection between bhakti yoga, the yoga of devotion, and karma yoga, the yoga of action and selfless service. He can accomplish anything because of the purity of his love for God. When he repeats Rām's name, Hanuman remembers who he *is*, and when he does things in Rām's name, nothing can stand in his way. Serving as Hanuman serves is a way of making your entire life an offering, an act of devotion. For Hanuman, each action is an opportunity to place a flower at the feet of Rām, the Beloved.

Maharaj-ji had us learn the "Hanuman Chalisa," forty verses in praise of Hanuman. The opening of the "Hanuman Chalisa" (see the invocation on page vi) inspired the title of this book. Krishna Das, who has helped spread the Chalisa in the West, says, "Chanting the Chalisa is a powerful way . . . to enter into the flow of Love and Grace. In the Chalisa, we bow to the great beauty, strength, and devotion that Hanuman embodies; we also begin to bow to that place in ourselves. The Chalisa inspires us to make the mirror of our heart as clean as Hanuman's so that we can become aware of the great beauty and love that lives within us as our own true nature."

Maharaj-ji said Hanuman is the breath of Rām.

Chapter 3

Karma Yoga, Living in the World

ONCE YOU GET that first glimpse of living Spirit, once your heart opens even for a moment to unconditional love, everything in your life becomes grist for the mill of your awakening. That awakening is from ego consciousness, your limited self, to the Self, the universal Spirit present in each of us, the God consciousness. It's such grace to share this path of the heart together.

Although I went through a major transformation on my journey, that's not how the journey goes for everyone, nor is rapid transformation necessary. For many people, their inner transformation occurs through subtle changes over long periods of time. In any case, it is a fallacy to think you'll get closer to God by changing the outer form of your life, by leaving your partner or changing your job or moving to another place, by growing your hair or cutting your hair or giving up your material possessions.

It is not the outer form that changes; it is the nature of the inner being that fills the form. If you're a lawyer, you go on being a lawyer, but you begin to use being a lawyer as a way of coming to God. One form is no more spiritual than any other. The essential work of developing a spiritual consciousness is quieting the mind and opening the heart.

YOUR KARMA IS YOUR DHARMA

The game of enlightenment starts from exactly where you are in your life at this moment. It's not about rejecting or walking away from any part of your life. The game is to bring all of your life into harmony at every level, to act according to dharma, the law of the universe, truth, how it all *is*.

Your karma is what you are given to do in your life, based on past actions. Making a spiritual practice out of your karma, using it to go to God, is what brings karma into dharma, life into harmony with the spirit. From a spiritual standpoint, the intent and the manner of doing something are more important than the act itself. When you bring all of your life into harmony at every level, you act in accord with dharma. Another way to say it is you're doing God's will.

All forms of yoga are ways of coming into union with God. Karma yoga is putting all the activity of your life—work, relationships, service—toward consummating that union. How you go about your work in the world determines whether your work is a vehicle for your spiritual awakening or for getting more caught in *maya,* increasing the illusion of separation. Karma yoga uses selfless action and service as a way of bringing your life into harmony with the One.

In the Bhagavad Gita, Krishna tells Arjuna to do what he does, but to offer the fruits of his actions to him, to Krishna, to God. To use your daily life and work as a conscious spiritual path means relinquishing your attachment to the fruits of the actions, to how they come out. Instead of doing it for a reward or a result, you do your work as an offering, out of love for God. Through love for God, your work becomes an expression of devotion, of bhakti.

Loving service to others is also a way of offering your work to God. In the *Ramayana,* Hanuman expresses his devotion through his service to Rām. Hanuman exemplifies that combination of bhakti (devotion) and karma yoga (service). Hanuman personifies Khalil Gibran's statement, "Work is love made visible." Like Hanuman, you serve others as a way of honoring

God. It's an attitude you develop, an attitude of offering. Every action you perform, you offer as selfless service, *"seva"* in Sanskrit. In the same vein, Christ says about service, "What you do for the least of my brothers and sisters you do for me."

Seva doesn't have ego in it; it's all soul. Any action can be seva. Everything you do—cooking, working, gardening—is an act you can offer to God. Offering your work and all your actions to God takes daily life out of the realm of ego and into the higher Self. Karma yoga is a great practice, especially for us Westerners who are so addicted to *doing,* because it opens us to *being* even while we're *doing.* Letting go of the doer lightens your load. It's not even your load any more. "Not my will, but Thy Will."

I slept and dreamt that life was joy.
I awoke and saw that life was service.
I acted and behold, service was joy.
RABINDRANATH TAGORE

Find someone or something that needs help, and help out. Work on yourself to make it a conscious act of seva. Gandhi said, "The act that you do may seem very insignificant, but it's important that you do it."

Another term for karma yoga is "right action." In the West the concept of right action is a difficult one to hear because it runs counter to our achievement and goal-oriented culture. In India, they have a very deep sense of doing one's dharma. From that view, it's natural to attune yourself to be in harmony with the laws of the universe. Your life is the part you play. You go from being the star of your own show to becoming an actor in the divine play.

That Bhagavad Gita instruction to be unattached to the fruits of your actions is the key. If you are a parent raising a child, don't get attached to the act of raising the child. That doesn't mean you're not a loving, active parent. Your job is to love and nurture, feed and clothe, take care and guard the safety of the child, and guide him or her with your moral compass. But how the child turns out is how the child turns out. Ultimately he or she is not *your* child; who they turn out to be is up to God and their own karma.

Your *attachment,* your clinging to how the child is going to turn out, affects every aspect of how you parent. A lot of our anxiety comes because we are attached to how a child is supposed to come out—smart, successful, creative, whatever it is we want for our child. Of course, you parent your child as impeccably as you can. "Parent" is your role to play because that is your dharma, and naturally you become immersed in your role in life. But it is also important to remember you're a *soul* playing a *role.* Who your child *is* and who you *are* are not roles.

As a conscious being, you do all you can to live in your soul and to create a space for others to be in their soul too. But you do so without trying to change the existing karma. You don't need to change your karma, only your attachment to it. Attachment is what keeps you stuck in your limited reality. Your attachment, wishing your loved ones to be different than they are, keeps them the same. Just allow them to be the way they are and love them. Then they may change. But it's not up to you. Samuel Johnson said, "He who has so little knowledge of human nature, as to seek happiness by changing anything but his own disposition, will waste his life in fruitless efforts."

Just keep working on yourself until you are radiating love for each of the beings in your life. When you are radiating love, then everybody else is free to give up their stuff when they're ready to give it up. Like a skillful gardener, you create a space for people to grow when they're ready to grow. As a parent you create the garden for a child to grow (that's why they call it kindergarten), but you don't grow the flower. You cultivate and fertilize the earth and keep it weeded and moist, and then the flower grows naturally.

WITNESSING YOUR OWN MELLOW DRAMA

The essence of karma yoga is to free yourself from attachments to the events of your life, to stop creating more karma that gets you more stuck, and to get free of your existing karma. The minute your awareness grasps at anything, whether through attraction or aversion, you create karma from that link between awareness and the acts (or thoughts or emotions) that follow from the desire or the aversion. Action arising from awareness not identified with attraction or aversion creates no karma. Karma is the residual effect of an attached act. No attachment, no karma.

The Great Way is not difficult
for those not attached to preferences.
When neither love nor hate arises
all is clear and undisguised.
Separate by the smallest amount, however
and you are as far from it as heaven is from earth.

If you wish to know the truth,
then hold to no opinions for or against anything.
To set up what you like against what you dislike
is the disease of the mind.

When the fundamental nature of things is not recognized
the mind's essential peace is disturbed to no avail.
. . .
When you try to stop activity to achieve quietude
your very effort fills you with activity.
. . .
Do not remain in a dualistic state
avoid such easy habits carefully.
If you attach even to a trace
of this and that, of right and wrong,
the Mind-essence will be lost in confusion.
Although all dualities arise from the One,
do not be attached even to ideas of this One.

When the mind exists undisturbed in the Way,
there is no objection to anything in the world,
and when there is no objection to anything,
things cease to be—in the old way.
SENG-TS'AN, FROM *HSIN-HSIN MING, VERSES ON THE FAITH-MIND,*
TRANSLATED BY RICHARD B. CLARKE

One way to get free of attachment is to cultivate the witness consciousness, to become a neutral observer of your own life. The witness place inside you is simple awareness, the part of you that is aware of everything—just noticing, watching, not judging, just being present, being here now.

The witness is actually another level of consciousness. The witness coexists alongside your normal consciousness as another layer of awareness, as the part of you that is awakening. Humans have this unique ability to be in two states of consciousness at once. Witnessing yourself is like directing the beam of a flashlight back at itself. In any experience—sensory, emotional, or conceptual—there's the experience, the sensory or emotional or thought data, and there's your awareness of it. That's the witness, the awareness, and you can cultivate that awareness in the garden of your being.

The witness is your awareness of your own thoughts, feelings, and emotions. Witnessing is like waking up in the morning and then looking in the mirror and noticing yourself—not judging or criticizing, just neutrally observing the quality of being awake. That process of stepping back takes you out of being submerged in your experiences and thoughts and sensory input and into self-awareness.

Along with that self-awareness comes the subtle joy of just being here, alive, enjoying being present in this moment. Eventually, floating in that subjective awareness, the objects of awareness dissolve, and you will come into the spiritual Self, the Atmān, which is pure consciousness, joy, compassion, the One.

The witness is your centering device. It guides the work you do on yourself. Once you understand that there is a place in you that is not attached, you can extricate yourself from attachments. Pretty much everything we notice in the universe is a reflection of our attachments.

Jesus warned us, "Lay not up for yourselves treasures upon earth, where moth and rust doth corrupt . . . For where your treasure is, there will your heart be also." Desire creates your universe; that's just the way it works. So your first job is to work on yourself. The greatest thing you can do for another human being is to get your own house in order and find your true spiritual heart.

After meditating for some years, I began to see the patterns of my own behavior. As you quiet your mind, you begin to see the nature of your own resistance, your stuckness, more clearly. You see the mental struggles, inner dialogues, self-narrations, the ways you procrastinate or resist life changes. Don't try to change the patterns; just notice them. As you cultivate the witness, things change. You don't have to change them. When you're being here now, in loving awareness, things just change.

By cultivating the witness consciousness, you move your identification from your ego to your soul. Your soul is in your spiritual heart. The soul witnesses the incarnation. If you stay in the witness, your soul witnesses your feelings, your desires, your experiences, not identifying with those desires or attitudes or any of those things. Then you can just watch the show. Sit back from your ego and your other thoughts and just watch the show of your incarnation like a movie, enjoying the characters and loving the melodrama. It turns out how it turns out. I like to sit back with my guru inside my heart. He is a loving and compassionate, peaceful and wise soul friend. You also can have a soul friend—inside yourself—a guru or a good spiritual friend to keep you oriented toward God.

Think of the witness as your inner guru, silently illuminating the workings of your mind. There is this quiet place, this conscious entity that's hanging around and showing you, "Oh, you just got uptight." Not judging, as in, "You're such a failure, you fool. You got uptight again," but just, "OK, you got uptight again. How interesting!"

The quickest way to get through your stuff is to learn to listen to that place inside. The inner guru is always there for you once you recognize it. You have to honor your own path and be able to trust that there is a place in you that knows what is best. There is a tendency to look to others for guidance, but really only you know what is suitable for you. Trust your intuitive heart. The Quakers call it the still, small voice within. When it speaks, listen. If, as you listen to your heart's intuition, it feels right to do something, do it.

Witnessing is a doorway to living in your spiritual heart, your soul awareness. The more you listen to your internal witness, the more you stop living by other people's judgments and expectations. You start doing what you need to do. In trying to decide what to do with your life, listen to your heart. The more you live in your spiritual heart, the more you see yourself and others from the soul perspective. Seeing things as a soul changes everything. The program is much farther out than you think. I never thought I'd be a yogi.

Each of us has our own unique karmic predicament, our own unique work to do. The predicament is that there is nowhere to stand, because our identification with the person who has the karma is changing too. As you develop the witness and identify more with your spiritual heart, karma just *is*. As you awaken, you realize that personal karma is just another illusion. The illusion is that this is the only reality. The witness helps you to see that there are choices, different ways to perceive reality.

When you are pouring morning tea or pouring the water into the coffeemaker for your family, is that all it is? Or is it God pouring God into God to serve God? Always choose what you feel is most at one with the Way of things, the Tao, your dharma.

IT'S ALL IN THE FAMILY

Back in the '70s we put out a boxed set of records called *Love, Serve, Remember.* It was a really nice box, with six records and a beautiful booklet with text and photos and drawings. My father, the lawyer and CEO, looked at it and said, "This is pretty good. How much do you sell it for?" I told him we sold it for just a little more than it cost to produce. He said, "You know, you could charge much more for this. It's worth it, and you could make more money."

I asked Dad how much he charged Uncle Henry when he represented him in a legal matter. He replied, "Well, of course I didn't charge him anything. That's Uncle Henry. He's family." I said that was my dilemma too—I see everyone as Uncle Henry. The way I see it, we are all one family. Now, whether I can actually live so everybody is my family and we are all one depends on how trapped I am in my separateness, and whether I see others as "us" or as "them." Of course, how you see others starts with how you see yourself. Who you think you are is a matter of perspective. I like the story about a disreputable-looking Sufi named Nasrudin, who is attempting to do some business in a bank. The bank teller asks him if he can identify himself. He pulls out a mirror and says, "Yep, that's me."

Don't take your melodrama so seriously. Let's remember who we really are—that is, souls, not egos. The ego is *who you think you are.* Who you think you are will die with the body because it's part of this incarnation. But your soul, which has these qualities of deep wisdom and love and peace and joy, is just here, watching it all go by.

Again, karma yoga is not about renouncing external actions but about renouncing your attachment to them. We're really talking about giving up being the central character of your own melodrama, who you think you are and how you think it is. All this self-narration of the ego is what keeps your personal melodrama going.

Ego is neither good nor bad. The ego has a function. It is the vehicle through which you relate to the external world. But the ego is a collection of thoughts, and to the extent you identify with your thoughts, they keep you from being here now. Once you let go of the identification with your thoughts the melodrama goes on, but it's no longer *your* melodrama. Appreciate the experiences but don't get caught in them.

The art of spiritual growth has to do with how quickly you recognize attachments and how quickly you can release them. If you can admit that you can't see or hear clearly because of attachment, then the full wisdom of things will begin to shine through. As long as you have some desire about how you think it ought to be, you can't hear how it *is.*

A Zen story about a monk living in a monastery in the hills above a town exemplifies life without attachment. A local girl got pregnant by a fisherman, but she didn't want to get the fisherman in trouble, so she said the monk on the hill was the father. The townspeople went up to the monastery with torches, and they knocked on the gate. The monk opened the gate, and they said, "This is your baby. You must raise it." The monk said, "Aahh, so." And he took the baby and closed the gates. Nine years later, the girl was dying but didn't want to die without confessing this terrible injustice, so she told the people. They were mortified, and they went rushing up and knocked on the gate. The monk opened the gate, and they said, "We're terribly sorry. It wasn't your son. We've come to relieve you of this responsibility." And he said, "Aahh, so."

RELATIONSHIPS AND EMOTIONS

From the soul's point of view, you come to appreciate that each one of us is living out his or her own karma. We interact together, and those interactions are the grist for each other's mill of awakening. From a personality point of view, you develop judgment, but from the soul's point of view, you develop appreciation. This shift from judging to appreciating—to appreciating yourself and what your karmic predicament is, and who other beings are with their own karma—brings everything into a simple loving awareness. To be free means to open your heart and your being to the fullness of who you are, because only when you are resting in the place of unity can you truly honor and appreciate others and the incredible diversity of the universe.

When I perform a wedding ceremony, the image I invoke is of a triangle formed by the two partners and this third force, which is the shared love that unites and surrounds them both. In the yoga of relationship, two people come together to find that shared love but continue to dance as two. In that union, both people are separate and yet not separate. Their relationship feeds both their unique individuality and their unity of consciousness. Love can open the way to surrendering into oneness. It gets extraordinarily beautiful when there's no more "me" and "you," and it becomes just "us."

Taken to a deeper level, when compassion is fully developed, you are not looking at others as "them." You're listening and experiencing and letting that intuitive part of you merge with the other person, and you're feeling their pain or joy or hope or fear in yourself. Then it's no longer "us" and "them"; it's just "us." Practice this in your relationships with others.

At a certain point, you realize that you see only the projections of your own mind. The play of phenomena is a projection of the spirit. The projections are your karma, your curriculum for this incarnation. Everything that's happening to you is a teaching designed to burn out your stuff, your attachments. Your humanity and all your desires are not some kind of error. They're integral parts of the journey.

One way of getting to this place of compassionate action is by honoring others and being patient. Look at the people you don't like and see them as an exercise for you to open your spiritual heart and to develop your compassion. The quieter you are, the more you hear the true nature of compassion. The intuitive compassionate heart is the doorway to our unity.

This story from Aikido master Terry Dobson is one of my favorites because it shows how to bring about harmony by embracing conflict with compassion and understanding:

> The train clanked and rattled through the suburbs of Tokyo on a drowsy spring afternoon. Our car was comparatively empty, a few housewives with their kids in tow, some old folks going shopping. I gazed absently at the drab houses and dusty hedgerows.
>
> At one station the doors opened and suddenly the afternoon quiet was shattered by a man bellowing violent, incomprehensible curses. The man staggered into our car. He wore laborer's clothing and he was big, drunk, and dirty. Screaming, he swung at a woman holding a baby. The blow sent her spinning into the laps of an elderly couple. It was a miracle the baby was unharmed. Terrified, the couple jumped up and scrambled toward the end of the car. The laborer aimed a kick at the retreating back of the old woman but missed as she scuttled to safety. This so enraged the drunk that he grabbed the metal pole in the center of the car and tried to wrench it out of its stanchion. I could see that one of his hands was cut and bleeding. The train lurched ahead, the passengers frozen with fear. I stood up.
>
> I was young then, some twenty years ago, and in pretty good shape. I had been putting in a solid eight hours of aikido training every day for the past three years. I liked to throw and grapple. I thought I was tough. The trouble was, my martial skill was

untested in actual combat. As students of aikido, we were not allowed to fight. Aikido, my teacher had said again and again, is the art of reconciliation. Whoever has the mind to fight has broken his connection to the universe. If you try to dominate people, you are already defeated. We study how to resolve conflict, not how to start it.

I listened to his words. I tried so hard. I even went so far as to cross the street to avoid the kids, the pinball punks who lounged around the train station. My forbearance exalted me. I was both tough and holy. In my heart, however, I wanted an absolutely legitimate opportunity whereby I might save the innocent by destroying the guilty. This is it, I said to myself, as I stood up. People are in danger. If I don't do something fast, somebody will probably get hurt.

Seeing me stand up the drunk recognized the chance to focus his rage. "Ah ha!" he roared. "A foreigner! You need a lesson in Japanese manners." I held on lightly to the commuter strap overhead and gave him a slow look of disgust and dismissal. I planned to take this turkey apart but he had to make the first move. I wanted him mad so I pursed my lips and blew him an insolent kiss. "All right," he hollered, "You're going to get a lesson." He gathered himself for a rush at me.

A fraction of a second before he could move, someone shouted "Hey!" It was ear-splitting. I remember the strangely joyous, lilting quality of it as though you and a friend had been searching diligently for something and he had suddenly stumbled upon it—"Hey!" I wheeled to my left, the drunk spun to his right.

We both stared down at a little old Japanese man. He must have been well into his seventies, this tiny gentleman, sitting there immaculate in his kimono. He took no notice of me but beamed delightedly at the laborer as though he had a most important, most welcome secret to share. "Come here," the old man said in an easy vernacular, beckoning to the drunk. "Come here and talk with me." He waved his hand lightly. The big man followed as if on a string. He planted his feet belligerently in front of the old gentleman and roared above the clacking wheels. "Why the hell should I talk to you?"

The drunk now had his back to me. If his elbow moved so much as a millimeter I'd drop him in his socks. The old man continued to beam at the laborer. "Whatcha been drinkin?" he asked, his eyes sparkling with interest. "I've been drinking sake," the laborer bellowed back, "and it's none of your business." Flecks of spittle spattered the old man. "Oh, that's wonderful," the old man said, "absolutely wonderful. You see I love sake too. Every night me and my wife, she's seventy-six you know, we warm up a little bottle of sake and we take it out in the garden and we sit on our old wooden bench and we watch the sun go down and we look to see how our persimmon tree is doing. My great-grandfather planted that tree and we worry about whether it will recover from those ice storms we had last winter. Our tree has done better than I expected though, especially when you consider the poor quality of the soil. It is gratifying to watch when we take our sake and go out to enjoy the evening even when it rains." He looked up at the laborer, his eyes twinkling.

As he struggled to follow the old man's conversation, the drunk's face began to soften. His fists slowly unclenched. "Yeah," he said, "I love persimmons too." His voice trailed off. "Yes," said the old man, smiling, "and I am sure you have a wonderful wife." "Nah. My wife died." Very gently, swaying with the motion of the train, the big man began to sob. "I don't got no wife. I don't got no home. I don't got no job. I'm so ashamed of myself." Tears rolled down his cheeks. A spasm of despair rippled through his body.

There I was standing in my well-scrubbed youthful innocence, my make-this-world-safe-for-democracy righteousness. I suddenly felt dirtier than he was. The train arrived at my stop. As the door opened, I heard the old man cluck sympathetically. "My, my," he

said, "that is a difficult predicament. Sit down here and tell me
about it." I turned my head for one last look. The laborer was
sprawled on the seat, his head in the old man's lap. The old man
was softly stroking the filthy matted hair. As the train pulled away,
I sat down on a bench. What I had wanted to do with muscle had
been accomplished with kind words. I had just seen aikido tried in
combat, and the essence of it was love.

You and I are in training to become conscious, compassionate beings, in
the truest and deepest sense. Become an instrument of joy, an instrument
of equanimity, an instrument of presence, an instrument of love, an instrument of availability, and at the same moment absolutely quiet. Since we
all spend so much time in our relationships, why not turn them into a
yoga for getting free? Living a spiritual life is a strategy for working on
yourself for the benefit of all beings. That's another way of saying that the
optimum thing you can do for someone else is to work on yourself—not
out of some idealistic sense of altruism, but because getting to oneness for
yourself means resolving your sense of separateness to where we're all family.

Use every situation you have with other people as a vehicle to work on
yourself. See where you get stuck, where you push, where you grab, where
you judge, where you do all the other stuff. Use your life experiences as
your curriculum.

When I look at relationships, my own and others, I see a whole range of
reasons we get together and ways we interact. Some are transactional, but
the deeper impulse of every human relationship is to evoke the love and
oneness that unites us. But what actually happens is that many relationships reinforce our separateness because of our misperception of ourselves
as separate beings, and because of our desire systems, which are based on
separateness or ego. Relationships only work in a spiritual sense when you
and I really see that we are one.

Relationships and emotions can reinforce our separateness, or they can
be grist for the mill of awakening. When it comes to love relationships we
are like bees looking for a flower. The predicament is that the emotional

power of loving somebody can get you so caught in the interpersonal melodrama that you can't get beyond the emotion. The problem with interpersonal love is that you are dependent on the other person to reflect love back to you. That's part of the illusion of separateness. The reality is that love is a state of being that comes from within.

The only thing you really ever have to offer another person is your own state of being. When you're not entrapped by another person's appearance or behavior, you can see behind all that to a deeper level of their being because your mind has tuned itself; you've shifted your focus just that little bit to see their soul. That soul quality is love.

When I was growing up, I used to be somebody. We were all in somebody training in those days. You become somebody, and then you tell everybody who you are. You hand out business cards, and you say, "How do you do? I am Somebody, and I do such and such." Everybody is very important and special, and each person assesses how much more important they are than everybody else. We were all in that training.

I became somebody because my parents wanted me to be special and my educators wanted me to be special, and they trained me how to do that. It's called ego structuring. I really made it. I was really somebody. My parents were proud of me. I could look in their eyes and see pride and appreciation. That part was very gratifying.

The only problem was, inside I felt lousy. I felt like somehow I should be happy. But I wasn't. I thought, "Well, happiness isn't everything, is it? As long as I am what everyone wants me to be, isn't that enough?" But it wasn't, and I felt very weird.

There is a story I've told many times that describes that feeling of weirdness. A man wanted to have a suit made. So he went to the best tailor in town, who was named Zumbach. Zumbach took his measurements and ordered the best material.

The man went in for the final fitting, and he put on the suit. One sleeve was two inches longer than the other. He said, "Zumbach, I don't want to complain. It's a beautiful suit. But this sleeve is two inches longer than that sleeve." Zumbach looked affronted. He said, "There's nothing wrong with the suit. It's the way you are standing." And he pushed one of the man's shoulders down and the other one up, and he said, "See, if you stand like that it fits perfectly."

The fellow looked in the mirror again, and there was all this loose material behind the collar. He said, "Zumbach, what's all this material sticking out?" Zumbach said, "There is nothing wrong with that suit. It's the way you are standing." And he pushed in the man's chin and made him hunch his shoulders. "See, it's perfect."

Finally the suit was fitting perfectly, and the man left. He was walking to the bus in his new, perfectly fitting suit, and somebody came up to him and said, "What a beautiful suit! I bet Zumbach the tailor made it."

The man said, "How did you know?"

"Because only a tailor of Zumbach's skill could make a suit fit so perfectly on somebody as crippled as you are."

Well, that was what I felt like. Everybody kept telling me what a beautiful suit I was wearing, but I felt like I was in Zumbach's suit.

Wearing Zumbach's suit is sort of what you feel like in some relationships. When you take off the suit and start to see behind the veils, it's as if you're looking at someone and saying, "Are you here? I'm here. Here we are. Far out!"

If somebody at work is a problem for you, they're not the one who needs to change. If someone is a problem for you, it's you who needs to change. If you feel they're causing you trouble, that's your problem. It's on you. Your job is to clear yourself.

If they're creating a problem for themselves, that's their karma. When Christ was being crucified and he said, "Forgive them, for they know not what they do," he was trying to help others out of being a problem for themselves. They weren't a problem for him, because he was clear.

Ideally you clear yourself right in the situation, but often it's too sticky and you can't do it. Step back then and do the practices you do in the morning and evening or on weekends to stay clear. Do the stuff that quiets you down inside.

Next time you go into that work situation, you may lose it again. Just go home and see how you lost it, examine it. You go in the next day and lose it again. You start keeping a diary of, "How did I lose it today?" Then you go and do it again. After a while, when you're starting to lose it, you don't buy in so much. You start to watch the mechanics of what it is that makes you lose it all the time. When you get to the point of seeing stuff as it's actually happening, the tendrils of attachment will begin to loosen.

If you don't appreciate me, that's your problem. If I need your love or your approval, then it's my problem. Then my needs are giving you power over me. But it's not your power—it's the power of my desire system. The power other people have to shake you out of your equanimity and love and consciousness has to do with your own attachments and the clinging of your mind.

This is where your work is on yourself, where you need to meditate more, where you need to reflect more, where you need a deeper philosophical framework. It's where you need to cultivate the witness more. It's where you need to practice opening your heart more in circumstances that aren't optimum or easy. This is your work. You were given a heavy curriculum, a full course load. This is it. There's no blame; you're not being graded. It's just what's on your plate at this moment.

Using relationships as a vehicle to freedom means we have to learn to *listen*—listen to each person at each level of their being. The art of listening comes from a quiet mind and an open heart. Listening uses all of your senses, and it is a subtle skill. Listen, just listen—not only with the ear, but also with your being. Your being becomes the instrument of listening. Your sensing mechanisms in life are not just your ears, eyes, skin, and analytic mind. It's something deeper, some intuitive quality of knowing. With all of your being, you become an antenna to the nature of another person. Then for the relationship to remain as living spirit, one of the best ingredients to put into the stew is truth.

TRUTH WILL SET YOU FREE

Gandhi spent his life in what he called "experiments in truth," just learning how to be truthful. He said, "Only God knows absolute Truth," and further, that he, being human, knew only relative truth, and that his understanding of it changed from day to day. Gandhi said that his commitment was to truth, not to consistency. It is important to honor your own truth even though to other people you may appear to be inconsistent. In a speech to the Muslim world, President Barack Obama quoted from the Koran, "Be conscious of God and always speak the truth." Compassionate use of truth requires discriminating wisdom, which comes from awareness of God within.

For a long time I thought truth was expressed in words, but that's not always so. There are truths that are communicated only in silence. You have to know when to use words and when to use silence. There is a difference between paranoid silence and cosmic silence. Cosmic silence is a plane of consciousness that cannot be expressed in words. From that place, words are like a finger pointing at the moon. Silence is a luxury we can afford when we feel safe together in shared awareness.

When I went to India for the second time, I brought Maharaj-ji a copy of the book *Be Here Now*. I didn't hear anything for a while, then one day he called me up to where he was sitting and said, "You're printing lies in this book."

I said, "Oh no, Maharaj-ji. Everything in the book is true."

He said, "It says here that Hari Dass Baba went into the jungle when he was eight years old." (You may recall that Hari Dass Baba was assigned by Maharaj-ji to teach me yoga.) Maharaj-ji said, "He didn't go into the jungle when he was eight years old. He worked in the Forestry Department until 1962."

Then he called a man over and asked, "What do you do?"

The man said, "I am the head of the Forestry Department."

Maharaj-ji said, "Do you know Hari Dass Baba?"

He said, "Oh yes, he worked for me until 1962."

Maharaj-ji said, "OK, go."

Then in similar fashion he showed me a couple of more fallacies in two more paragraphs, and he said, "Why did you write that?"

I said, "Well, somebody told me all that stuff. I don't know who told it to me, but somebody did, and it was somebody around you. And I believed it because it was all coming with love."

He said, "Are you so simple that you believe everything everybody tells you?"

Hari Dass Baba was a beautiful silent yogi, and he was just being who he was. Maybe I'd developed this trip about him and listened to it because I wanted my teacher to be special.

Maharaj-ji said, "Whatever the reason, it's a lie. What are you going to do about it?"

I said, "Well Maharaj-ji, I'll change it. Eighty thousand copies are already distributed, and I can't call them back. But the second printing is coming up, and I will change it then."

I sent a telegram to the Lama Foundation, which was printing the book in Albuquerque. I told them to please delete the two paragraphs about Hari Dass Baba in the next printing. Steve Durkee, the then-head of Lama who is now called Nur al Din, wrote back and said, "It can't be done now. I was just in Albuquerque"—which is a couple of hundred miles from Lama, where there's no phone—"I told them to go ahead and print it, and they were going to press that day." It was the pre-Christmas rush, and it was probably already printed. Steve said, "I received your telegram too late. We will change it in the third edition, which will be printed in three months."

I went back to my guru and I said, "Maharaj-ji, I can't change it until the next edition. To change it now would cost at least $10,000. We would have to throw away the whole printing."

He looked at me and he said, "Do it now." And he said, "Money and truth have nothing to do with one another."

I went back and cabled Lama again and said, "Forget the expense. Maharaj-ji says change it now. It's his book."

A cable came back from Steve saying, "The most remarkable thing happened. The day your cable came telling us to change it anyway, a note came from the printing company. When they put the job on the press, one of the plates was damaged. That page included a photo of Maharaj-ji, and when they went to the file to find the original, that particular picture was missing. It was the only thing missing. So they took the whole job off the press and wrote for further instructions."

Money and truth have nothing to do with one another. Maharaj-ji was playing with the book and the printer and my mind.

The Tao Te Ching says, "Truth waits for eyes unclouded by longing." Often we don't fully hear the truth because of our mind's clinging or attachment; we hear only the projections of our own desires. So again and again we make decisions that end up not being in the deepest harmony with the Tao, the Way of things. Working through an attachment means you have to work with that desire until you are no longer attached to that desire. The desire may still be there, but you are no longer attached to it.

When we see without attachment, truth becomes self-evident. When we are fully present in the moment, truth just *is*.

WORKING WITH YOUR EMOTIONS

One way to heal your emotional problems is to cultivate another part of your being, like the witness. Use the witness to cultivate awareness in dealing with emotions one by one. As the witness gets stronger, your emotional problems become less relevant to your existence.

By witnessing, you can divest emotions of their power. When you're deep in the psychological realm and you keep trying to work it out, you just keep investing in it. It's a bottomless well of stuff.

Witnessing will allow you to acknowledge the feelings and appreciate them as part of the human condition. That's the quickest way through an emotion: to acknowledge it, allow it to be, and release it, give it up. You can do that in a variety of ways. For example, you can use the body energy of hatha yoga to keep working out the chemical stuff and the tension that builds up in the body. Sometimes music helps, or just becoming aware of your breath. Just keep letting go and letting go. Singing to God—as in the practice known as kirtan—can give rise to ecstatic states that have the power to free you from your personal emotional melodramas.

As your spiritual practice gets stronger, you are able to see your emotional stuff before it gets so overloaded and invested with adrenalin. You no longer let it get that intense. If those feelings get out of control, the best thing to do is to sit quietly. Let them pass. Bhagavan Das once said to me,

"Emotions are like waves. Watch them disappear in the distance on the vast calm ocean."

That capacity to dwell in the witness makes all the emotional stuff and stresses of life much lighter. The art, as I understand it, is to cultivate these other planes of consciousness, and then you no longer have to push the stuff away because it falls into perspective. It's as if you just shift your focus and see it from outside of yourself, so you are no longer identified with the way you were thinking. Einstein said, "The significant problems we have cannot be solved at the same level of thinking with which we created them."

On the devotional path, you can change levels by offering an emotion to God or your guru as a way to give it up. "Here, you take it. I offer it to you." And by appreciating your own humanity: "Yeah, here I am. I just lost it again. Ah, so. Right. OK." It's the ability to see it without denying it. "I'm upset. Far out. Here we are again." It is like talking with God and saying, "Look how deliciously human I am."

When I studied people's personalities in psychology, I saw that at the root of almost every problem was a feeling of inadequacy or not-enoughness. These are the seed components in personality structure. Understand these issues and see that you're subject to that pathology just like everyone else. That wisdom leads to compassion and love for yourself and others.

Go behind your own polarities too—not to "I am good" or "I am loveable," but go behind them to "I am." "I am" includes the fact that I do beautiful things and I do crappy things. And I am. As you start to rest in the space of "I am," you begin to feel emotions from a different perspective and become impeccable in the way you play the game. Loving those emotions helps to release them.

When you hunger for love, that is the longing to come home, to be at peace, to feel at one with the universe, where lover and Beloved merge. It's a place to *be* fully in the moment, to feel completely fulfilled, to just *be* in love.

I'D RATHER *BE* THAN BE RIGHT

Watch how your mind judges. Judgment comes, in part, out of your own fear. You judge other people because you're not comfortable in your own being.

By judging, you find out where you stand in relation to other people. The judging mind is very divisive. It separates. Separation closes your heart. If you close your heart to someone, you are perpetuating your suffering and theirs. Shifting out of judgment means learning to appreciate your predicament and their predicament with an open heart instead of judging. Then you can allow yourself and others to just be, without separation.

The only game in town is the game of being, which includes both highs and lows. Every time you push something away, it remains there. The pile under the rug gets very big. Your lows turn out to be more interesting than your highs because they are showing you where you're not, where you have work to do.

You just say, "Thank you for the teaching." You don't have to judge another being. You just have to work on yourself.

When somebody provokes your anger, the only reason you get angry is because you're holding on to how you think something is supposed to be. You're denying how it is. Then you see it's the expectations of your own mind that are creating your own hell. When you get frustrated because something isn't the way you thought it would be, examine the way you thought, not just the thing that frustrates you. You'll see that a lot of your emotional suffering is created by your models of how you think the universe should be and your inability to allow it to be as it is.

Maharaj-ji told me to love everyone. "Love everyone, there is only one. *Sub ek*—it's all one, just love everyone. See God everywhere. Just love everyone. Don't get angry. Ram Dass, don't get angry. Love everyone, tell the truth, love everyone, don't get angry."

You know, when people say things like that to you, you say, "Yeah, sure, right, absolutely!" And it sort of goes through you like Chinese food because you've been told that since you were a child.

I had just returned to India after two years as a holy man in the West. It had been too heavy a trip for me because I was still full of lust and greed and laziness. There were so many more pizzas I still had to eat, and it was hard to sneak in a pizza when somebody was always looking. Finally I had fled back to India, hoping to hide out in a cave until I could get my head together. But all the time in India, wherever I would go there were Western-ers wanting to hang out. Slowly I grew to hate them all. How could I go into a cave and get holy with forty Westerners?

After a year, except for a couple of weeks, I remained totally immersed in Western consciousness in the middle of India. We were all with Maharaj-ji, and finally I decided, "Well, he keeps saying tell the truth and don't get angry, but the truth is I am angry. I have spent too long outwardly pretend-ing I love everyone. Inside my mind is full of anger. The hypocrisy is driving me up the wall. Maharaj-ji said to tell the truth. I think for a change I will tell the truth, since I can't do both."

People would come to visit me in my room. They were lovely beings, and I would say, "Get the hell out of this room, you lazy bastard. You're too nice. You nauseate me." Pretty soon I had effectively alienated the entire group. They didn't want to take me seriously, but I was persistent. At that time I was doing a sadhana, a practice, where I didn't touch money. To get to the temple every day from town, we usually shared a bus or a taxi, and somebody would pay for me. But I was so mad at everybody that I couldn't be in the same space with them on the bus. So I walked to the temple, which took several hours.

One day I got there late, having walked, and I was really angry. Every-one was sitting in the courtyard across from Maharaj-ji eating the blessed food, the *prasad*. There was one leaf plate left for me. One of the guys I was particularly angry at brought the food over and put it down in front of me. I was so angry I picked it up and threw it at him. Maharaj-ji was watching all of this and called me over. "Ram Dass, is something trou-bling you?"

"Yes. I can't stand *adharma,* I can't stand impurities. I can't stand all those people, and I can't stand myself. I only love you. I hate everybody else."

At that point I started to wail—to just cry and cry as if all the anger in me was just pouring out of me. Maharaj-ji sent for some milk, and he was feeding me milk and patting me on the head and pulling my beard, and he was crying along with me. And then he looked at me and he said, "Love everyone and don't get angry."

I said to him, "Well, you told me to tell the truth, and the truth is I don't love everyone."

He leaned close to me—like nose to nose and eye to eye—and very fiercely he said, "Love everyone and tell the truth."

I started to say, "But . . . ," and at that point the whole rest of that sentence became self-evident to me. He was saying, "When you finish being who you think you are, this is who you will be." I was thinking I was somebody who couldn't love everyone and tell the truth. He was saying, "Well, when you give that one up, I am still here, and the game is very simple. Love everyone and tell the truth."

I looked across at the group of Westerners—after all, this was an order from my guru. I looked at this group of people I was so angry with, and now I could see there was a place in them I did love.

Then he said, "Go take food." I went over and started eating. I was still crying.

He called everybody over to him and said, "Ram Dass is a great saint, go touch his feet." That completely infuriated me.

Usually when you are angry with somebody, what you do is sit down and talk it out until everybody saves face. You know how that's done: "I was wrong, I'm sorry." "Well, that's good of you to say so . . ." The trouble was, he didn't say I should save face. He just said to love everyone and tell the truth. He was telling me to give it up.

I saw that the only reason I got angry was because I was holding on to how I thought it was supposed to be. So I cut some apples into pieces, and I went around and I looked each person in the eye. I couldn't feed them the piece of apple until I was free of the anger, because to give food with anger is like giving somebody poison. The vibration of anger gets transmitted along with the food. It's the opposite of healing. I looked each person in the eye, and I saw everything I was angry at. And it began to dissolve. I could feel that the only thing that was between us at this point was my pride. I just didn't want to give up my righteousness. But I saw in each case that I had to just shed it—just let it go until I could look into their eyes and just see my guru, see myself, see their soul. I had to let go of our individual differences. It took quite a long time because I had to give it up with each individual, and some took longer than others.

After that kind of teaching you might think that I don't get angry anymore. I do. But when I start to get angry, I see my predicament and how I'm getting caught in expectations and righteousness. Learning to give up anger has been a continuous process. When Maharaj-ji told me to love everyone and tell the truth, he also said, "Give up anger, and I'll help you with it." Maharaj-ji offered me a bargain: "You must polish the mirror free of anger to see God. If you give up a little anger each day, I will help you." This seemed to be a deal that was more than fair. I readily accepted. And he's been true to his end of the bargain. I found that his love helped to free me from my righteousness. Ultimately I would rather be free and in love than be right.

If you feel a sense of social responsibility, first of all keep working on yourself. Being peaceful yourself is the first step if you want to live in a peaceful universe.

Have you ever noticed how many angry people there are at peace rallies? Social action arouses righteousness. Righteousness ultimately starves you to death. If you want to be free more than you want to be right, you have to let go of righteousness, of being right.

That reminds me of a story. There's this Chinese boatman, and he hits another boat in the fog. He starts swearing at the other boatman. "You SOB! Why didn't you look where you were going?" Then the fog lifts for a moment, and he sees there is nobody in the other boat. And he feels like a fool.

Righteousness is roughly the same thing. Say, for instance, you hold a grudge against your father, and you talk to him in your mind as if he's there inside you. But he isn't there. Psychologically you *think* he is there, because you're identified with who you think *you* are, but once you begin to see this is all just a bunch of thoughts, your psychological father is just another set of empty phenomena. You are busy saying, "I forgive you, I forgive you," to that psychological father, but it's like saying "I forgive you" to a clock. There's nothing there. You're the same as the boatman.

There's no rush. Go on being right just as long as you can. You'll see that being right is actually a tight little box that is very constraining and not much fun to live in. Righteousness cuts you off from the flow of things. When I'm locked in a situation in a relationship with someone, it isn't that they have done something *to* me. They're just doing what they're doing. If I get caught up in judging, the responsibility lies with me, not with them. It becomes my work on myself. I often say, "I really apologize for whatever suffering I've caused you in this situation." We start to work from there. And after a while they will come forward and will examine themselves and say, "Well, maybe I was . . ." Our predicament is that our ego wants to be right in a world of people who don't understand how right we are.

There is a way of representing what is right, the dharma of the moment. But if you get emotionally attached to a model of how the world ought to be that excludes how human beings are, there's something wrong with where you're standing. You should be standing somewhere else. Getting lost in your emotional reactivity isn't where you want to be. Just allowing your humanity and that of others to be as it is, is the beginning of compassion.

We are in a human incarnation. We can't walk away. To walk in the dharma is also to hear other human beings.

FAITH, NO FEAR—NO FAITH, FEAR

As you tune into your own dharma, you become motivated to confront the places in yourself that keep you trapped. When there is fear, you aren't free. President Franklin Roosevelt said, "The only thing we have to fear is fear itself."

Fear is a protective mechanism in the sense that you experience free-floating anxiety about that which threatens you. Fear makes you want to hold on to familiar structure in your life. If you are busy identifying yourself as a separate entity, you fear the extinction of that being. When you are identified with your soul, there is no fear. The soul doesn't identify with the ending of the incarnation, which we think of as death.

Since meeting Maharaj-ji, I do not experience a fear of death as a real fear when I get into situations where death seems imminent. I don't have any of my earlier usual reactions of anxiety or fear, and yet I protect the temple that is my body, because it is the vehicle for my work. I don't protect it out of fear, because the fear of death seems somehow to have flown the coop somewhere along the way. The absence of that fear changes the nature of my daily experience. Now each day is just what it is.

When you experience fear, you are caught in your separateness, feeling cut off and vulnerable. When you're experiencing love, you're part of the unity of all things. Love is the antidote for fear because it goes to the place behind separateness. As you cultivate that unitive quality, the fear dissipates. As fear dissipates, you feel at home in the universe. If you stay in the soul, you will stay in love. It's not a concept or a belief. When you have faith, there's no fear—only love. True "faith" arises when you know that you are the soul, and that the soul *is* love.

Once, back in 1970, I was driving on the New York Thruway in a 1938 Buick limousine that I had converted into a camper. I was going very slowly because it was a very old car, driving with one hand on the steering wheel and doing my māla beads with the other—just hanging out with various forms of the Divine. I was holding the steering wheel with just enough consciousness to keep the car on the road. I was singing to Krishna, a radiant, blue incarnation of God who plays the flute. Krishna represents the seductive aspect of the Beloved. I was ecstatically hanging out with blue Krishna and driving along the New York Thruway when I noticed a blue, flashing light in my rearview mirror. I thought, "Krishna has come!"

There was enough of me focused on driving that I knew it was a state trooper. I pulled over, and he came up to the car window. He said, "May I see your license and registration?"

I was looking at him as Krishna, who had come to give me *darshan*. It was 1970. Wouldn't Krishna come as a state trooper? Christ came as a carpenter.

Krishna asked for my license. I would have given him anything; he could have my life, but all he wanted was my license and registration. So I gave him my license and registration, and it was like I was throwing flowers at the feet of God. I was looking at him with absolute love.

He went back to his police car, and he called home base. Then he came back, and he walked around the car, and he said, "What's in that box on the seat?"

I said, "They're mints. Would you like one?"

He said, "Well, the problem is you were driving too slowly on the thruway, and you'll have to drive off the thruway if you're going to drive that slowly."

I said, "Yes, absolutely." I was just looking at him with such love.

If you put yourself in the role of a state trooper, how often do you suppose they get looked at with unconditional love, especially when they're in uniform? So after he had finished all the deliberations, he didn't want to leave, but he had run out of state trooper-ness. So he stood there a minute, and then he said, "Great car you've got here!"

That allowed me to get out. And we could kick the tires and hit the fenders and say, "They don't make 'em now like they used to," and tell old car stories. Then we ran out of that. I could feel he still didn't want to leave. I mean, why would you want to leave if you're being unconditionally loved?

So finally he ran out of digressions. He knew he'd have to come clean that he's Krishna, so he said, "Be gone with you," which wasn't state trooper talk, but what the hell. As I got into the car and started to drive away, he was standing by his cruiser. I looked in the mirror and saw that he was waving at me.

Tell me, was that a state trooper or was that Krishna?

SPIRITUAL FAMILY AND FRIENDS

As these spiritual practices start to work, your reasons for being with people start to change, and who you want to be with changes too. Sometimes it's not easy, as longstanding relationships or jobs are discarded. Your old friends might find you a little dull because you've experienced a taste of a certain kind of truth—a deeper truth connected to a different quality of being. Social interactions that used to be engaging pale next to the attraction to the Beloved, and social life begins to seem surreal. Not everyone can "hear" the quality of the spiritual experience you are having. You are looking for God, for whatever form of the Beloved touches your heart. You are looking everywhere.

The poet-saint Kabir says:

Are you looking for me? I am in the next seat.
My shoulder is against yours.
You will not find me in stupas, not in Indian shrine rooms, nor in
synagogues, nor cathedrals:
not in masses, nor kirtans, not in legs winding around your own neck,
nor in eating nothing but vegetables.
When you really look for me, you will see me instantly—
You will find me in the tiniest house of time.
Kabir says, Student, tell me, what is God?
He is the breath inside the breath.

When you are first awakening and developing a spiritual perspective, satsang is especially supportive. Satsang is like having a spiritual family. Satsang is a community of truth seekers. It is a group of people with the shared awareness that there is a spiritual dimension to the universe. Goethe had this beautiful thought: "The world is so empty if one thinks only of mountains, rivers and cities; but to know someone here and there who thinks and feels with us, and who, though distant is close to us in spirit, this makes the earth for us an inhabited garden."

Once we get a taste of the freedom that comes with letting go of our stuff—anger, righteousness, jealousy, our need to be in control, the judging mind, to name just a few—we start to look at those things in new ways. That is the teaching of being in the moment. For someone who understands that this precious birth is an opportunity to awaken, is an opportunity to know God, all of life becomes an instrument for getting there—marriage, family, job, play, travel, all of it. You just spiritualize your life.

Christ said to be in the world but not of the world. You are simultaneously living your story line—keeping your ground, remembering your zip code—*and* having your awareness free and spacious, not caught in anything, just delighting in the richness of this timeless moment.

Chapter 4

Aging and Changing

IT WAS LATE EVENING. The station was closed, so I had to buy my ticket on the train. I had just turned sixty. When the conductor came by I said, "I'd like a senior ticket." I felt like I had when I was eighteen in New York and had gone to a bar with friends. With trepidation, because I was under the drinking age, I said to the bartender, "I'll have a beer." Now the conductor immediately made out a ticket for a senior citizen. I said, "Don't you want to see my ID?" He said, "No, it's OK." I was shocked.

Until I was about fifty, I thought of myself as a teenager. Around that time, I began to consider the possibility that I was an adult. I was busy being spiritual, and I thought age was rather uninteresting. After all, spiritual people are ageless, right?

Once I turned sixty, I decided I better see if there was any work I needed to do around aging. In past years, I was usually traveling on my birthday, so people couldn't give parties for me. This year I let friends know I wanted a birthday party because sixty is a big year. I had several parties. I kept busy becoming sixty for about six months.

One day I looked down at my hand, and I saw my father's hand. "That's a sixty-year-old hand," I thought. "With bones and blood vessels, wrinkles, and spots." I remembered this ad for Porcelana hand cream, which said, "They call these aging spots. I call them ugly." Now, isn't that an extraordinary way to create suffering? Another way to look at it is just, "They call these aging spots." And here we are.

I began to feel like maybe it was time to close things out rather than start new projects. Maybe I should write my last book or take off for six months a year. As I traveled, I found the airport corridors leading to the gates seemed to be getting longer. I was steeping myself in what it was like to be getting older, to slow down and honor the process.

At the same time I was savoring the feeling of aging, I began behaving in a somewhat bizarre manner. I realized I was trying to act younger, trying to accomplish things for which I was no longer in physical shape. I went bodysurfing in the South Pacific with a thirty-three-year-old friend. There I was, paddling in the waves of Tahiti, surrounded by fifteen- to twenty-year-olds, out there having fun. But I was struggling. I took a wrong turn and ended up getting pounded by a wave against a coral reef and cutting my legs. The young surfers looked at me with pity. I thought, "What the heck am I doing?"

My father used to recite a verse that came back to me in that moment:

It's not the crow's feet under your eyes that make you old,
Or the gray in your hair, I'm told.
But when your mind makes a contract your body can't fill,
You're over the hill, brother, you're over the hill.

Much of the suffering of aging comes from holding onto those memories of who we used to be. When I was sixty-three and writing a book on aging, I saw that I needed to be able to dance through this part of my life's curriculum without denial, without closing down to the suffering, but just watching the way my energies become less reliable, the way my patterns of life change. For instance, I now have to live more economically. I watch how society takes away my power as it makes me into a senior citizen.

But instead of struggling with every change of circumstance, it's just, "*Ah, another new moment!*"

CULTURAL ATTITUDES ON AGING

In the United States you might retire at fifty-five or sixty-five or maybe later. Medicare for health care begins at sixty-five, but other than starting to qualify for senior discounts, there's no clear rite of passage for becoming an elder or a senior, and you don't quite know what the cutoff is for being considered old.

Economic productivity and social roles cause so much stress in our society—this modern hunting tribe. In traditional hunting societies, the tribe has to keep moving, and when old people can't keep up, they tend to just be left behind. In terms of having a function, they're treated as irrelevant.

I am reminded of the story of an old Chinese man who retires. He is too old even to help the family work in the garden. One day the family is sitting on the porch, talking, and the old man's son thinks, "You know, he's so old. He just eats food. What good is he? Now it's time for him to be done." So he makes a wooden box, puts the box on the wheelbarrow, and rolls the wheelbarrow up to the porch and says, "Father, get in." The father gets into the box. The son puts the cover on the box and starts to wheel it toward the cliff. As he gets to the edge of the cliff, there's a knocking from inside the box. The father says, "Son, I understand what you're doing and why you're doing it, but may I suggest you just throw me over the cliff and save the box. Your children will need it later."

One thing that helped me avoid getting trapped in our Western, youth-biased model was that I traveled a lot. I was always surprised how different the feelings around aging were in other cultures. While I was in India, I saw a dear old friend in a village in the mountains. He said to me, "Ram Dass, you're looking so old. You're so gray!" My first reaction to that was my Western conditioning, "What an insult! God, that's terrible!" But when I quieted down, I heard the tone in which he spoke. He was saying it with great respect and affection. I had become a respected elder in that society. He was saying, "You've earned the respect due an elder. You're someone whose wisdom we can rely on and to whom we will listen."

The Vedic philosophy of India has four principle stages of life, or *ashramas*:

- To age 20, you are a student.
- From 20 to 40, you're a householder, raising children and earning money.
- From 40 to 60, when your children are grown, they take over your business, and you study philosophy, make pilgrimages, and do spiritual practice.
- From 60 on, you give up your responsibilities. You are free. Society supports you because it needs the wisdom you have to offer.

In cultures with extended-family structures, everybody has natural roles, and old people are honored and respected. They remain part of the family, and the old and young become wise fools together. It's all built into the system. But in our Western culture, we have an aging problem.

Western technology moves so fast that we quickly become outdated. The usefulness of our elders' wisdom becomes questionable. I tried to learn new computer programs, and I told myself old dogs *can* learn new tricks. But I don't know how many new tricks I want to learn. Maybe I will just choose to be outdated.

Let's at least recognize that we are living in a system that has gotten out of balance. You and I are paying the price for having grown up in a materially oriented society that values people in terms of their products, their achievements, and their ability to consume, instead of cultivating the quality of their being. The zeal for independence and individuality has alienated us not only from our deeper being, from family and community, but also from nature.

Being out of touch with nature, as many of us are, we overlook the cycles of cold and warm, of autumn leaves falling—the natural cycles of birth, fruition, harvest, winter's death, and the rebirth of spring. The cycles of nature give an intuitive, innate meaning to aging. And they give you a feeling of the appropriateness of time and place. If our old people feel empty of purpose, perhaps it is because our culture's vision for the end of life is lacking too.

DEALING WITH CHANGE

An older man is walking down the street, and he hears a voice saying, *"Psst, could you help me out?"*

He looks around, but he doesn't see anybody.

Again he hears, *"Psst, could you help me out?"*

He looks down, and there is a big frog. He's embarrassed—I mean, you don't talk to frogs. But he says, "Did you speak to me?"

And the frog says, "Yeah, could you help me out?"

"Well, what's the problem?"

"I'm under a curse. If you pick me up and kiss me, I will turn back into a beautiful maiden, and I will serve you and cook for you and warm your bed, and I will be everything you ever wanted."

The man stood there for a little while. Then he picked up the frog, and he put it in his pocket and walked on.

After a while the frog said, "Hey, you forgot to kiss me."

The man said, "You know, at my age I think it is more interesting to have a talking frog."

The nature of aging has to do with change. Old age trains you for change—change in your body, change in memory, change in your relationships, change in energy, change in your family and social role—all leading to death, which is the big change in our lives. You can see this last part of your life, the age stage, as a diminution. On the other hand, from a spiritual standpoint, many of these aspects are sensationally great. The clamor of the ego calms, your motivations become clear, and wisdom begins to come forth.

Wisdom is one thing in life that does not diminish with age. Wisdom is learning how to live in harmony with the world as it is in any given moment. One aspect of that wisdom is the deep understanding that we are all in the same boat. Out of that comes compassion—compassion for yourself, compassion for others, compassion for the world. Can you allow the changes and delight in them and look for the wisdom inherent in each change rather than resisting them?

Changing phenomena are endlessly wonderful and fascinating. But when who we think we are begins to change, the fascination turns into fear. Aging brings personal changes that are both physical and psychological. It's painful and confusing when the body doesn't do what it used to do, and starts to do a lot of things it didn't used to do.

Physical changes are endless, and if you're identified with your body, they can completely grab your consciousness. Whole Sunbelt colonies in places like St. Petersburg, Florida, or Phoenix, Arizona, are full of people sitting on benches reciting these changes to each other. They call them "organ recitals." You don't ask, "How are you?" unless you have the time to listen.

While you can hear how real that is for some people, just imagine sitting on those same benches with people like Albert Einstein, Pablo Picasso, Claude Monet, Marc Chagall, Bob Hope, Grandma Moses, or Margaret Mead. Can you imagine them having the same responses?

Part of how we deal with change depends on our perception. Perceptually, each of us is two beings, an ego and a soul, that function on different planes of consciousness. If we live predominantly in our soul, then the changes in the body are interesting, like changes in the weather.

Here's a way to think of perception. Suppose you have a little television receiver next to your eyes. Let's pretend the various planes of consciousness are channels on this television set. Most of us, most of the time in this culture, act as if we have a one- or two-channel set. We don't have cable or satellite TV with hundreds of channels. But maybe we've heard about cable, and we can at least acknowledge the existence of these other channels floating around in the room, even though we're not picking them up. We can't receive them because we don't know how to tune our receiver. That's basically what perception is about.

On channel one, when you look at another human being, you see the physical body: old, young, dark, light, fat, thin, and so on. Especially if you're obsessed with your own physical body, that's what you see when you look at the world: other people's physical bodies. That's the channel you're seeing. Youth, sex, fitness, fashion, beauty, sports—you know the programming.

Flip to channel two, and you're in the psychosocial realm. You see power, and you see happiness and sadness and neurosis. This is the therapy channel and the social role channel. Here, we are mothers and truck drivers and lawyers—all the different roles and identities, intricacies of character and interaction, all the social stuff. It's *As the World Turns,* a fascinating, never-ending soap opera that just goes on and on, episode after episode. Most people are happy with channel two. Maybe 98 percent of the people you meet are busy with these two channels all the time.

Now suppose you turn to yet another channel. This is the astral channel. Here you're seeing archetypes, the Jungian archetypes. You're dealing with what are called astral or mythic roles and mythic identities. It's the sort of place where you see people in their mythos rather than in their personality structures. You'd look at me, and you'd say, "He's an Aries. I just knew it," in the same way you'd know someone's a Sagittarius or a Leo. On this channel there are only twelve of us in various permutations.

But if you flip to the next channel, you go behind all those individual differences, and all you see is another soul, just like you. All the packaging is different, but inside the wrapping each one is another being just like you. That's when you say, "Are you in there? I'm in here. How'd you get in that one?" All of the personality stuff and the astral and mythic archetypes and the physical form—all of it is packaging. Inside, you see the individual spiritual entity.

Now, just for fun turn the channel once more. Here, you're looking at yourself looking at yourself—pure awareness looking at itself. And there's only one of it.

You try to live life in a way that is harmonious with what you know on these other planes of consciousness. That harmony is part of the wisdom that comes with age. Learning how to grow old is the masterwork of wisdom and one of the most difficult chapters in the great art of living.

One of the subtle traps of the ego, of the mind getting caught on channel one or two, is your concept of time, because aging has to do with time. But there is a part of you that is not in time, and finding that place and resting in it is a key part of the mystical journey. What you begin to see is that the spiritual journey is one of going deeper and deeper into your being, going behind the part of you that changes, to seek the part that does not change.

All the universe is but a sign to be read rightly. . . . War and peace, love and separation are hidden gateways to other worlds. . . . Let us not grow old still believing that truth is what most people see around them.
FROM THE RAMAYANA, WILLIAM BUCK

AGING GRACEFULLY

Here's the predicament: things change—my car gets old, my body gets old. The external changes are obvious. The harder and subtler task is to recognize that thoughts and feelings are also part of what changes.

As you age, some of those thoughts and feelings in your life will be traumatic because they counter the core model of who you think you are. As long as you identify with your thoughts and feelings, as long as you think those thoughts and feelings *are* you, they will be a source of suffering.

As you face the changes associated with aging, you can get trapped in a whole list of grim psychological possibilities: despair, depression, feelings of worthlessness, frustration, doubt, vulnerability, forgetfulness, irritability, loss of self-confidence, fear of the future, obsession with possessions, lack of meaning, loss of friends, fear of not having enough money, no one to touch, loss of power or influence, lack of focus and goals, to name just a few. Part of the psychological trap is your social support system, which also changes as you retire from your life's work. You may have to leave your home. You have less responsibility. Reward systems you worked so hard for don't reward you anymore. You may try to maintain psychological security by holding onto things as they are. But you never know.

There is a story of a farmer who had a horse that ran away. His neighbor came by and said, "Oh, that's terrible."

The farmer said, "You never know."

The next day the horse came back, and it was leading two other wild horses. The neighbor said, "That's wonderful."

And the farmer said, "You never know."

Later, his son was training one of the wild horses, and while riding the wild horse, he fell off and broke his leg. The neighbor came by and said, "That's terrible."

The farmer said, "You never know."

The Cossack army came through recruiting everybody, taking away all the able young men. They didn't take the farmer's son because he had a broken leg. The neighbor came by and said, "That's wonderful."

And the farmer said, "You never know."

And so it goes.

There is a spiritual model that will allow us to age gracefully instead of the old psychological model that is fearful and frightened. Martin Buber says, "To be old can be glorious if one has not unlearned what it means to begin."

Use the new uncertainty and negative feelings about aging as a wake-up call. Have compassion for yourself and allow yourself to open to the changes, and all the rest will follow.

In a Hallmark card, I found a poem about losing our mind. Forgetting is great because it's such fun to remember. But the greatest psychological fear we have is of losing our mind. This poem says:

Just a line to say I'm living, I'm not among the dead,
though I'm getting more forgetful and more mixed up in the head.
Sometimes I can't remember when I stand at the foot of the stair
if I must go up for something or if I've just come down from there.
And before the fridge so often my poor mind is full of doubt
have I just put food away or have I come to take some out. And there
are times when it is dark out with my night cap on my head
I don't know if I am retiring or just getting out of bed.

So if it is my turn to write you there is no need for getting sore.
I may think that I've written and don't want to be a bore.
Remember I do love you I wish you were here.
It's nearly mail time so I'll say goodbye dear.

There I stood beside the mailbox with my face so very red.
Instead of mailing you my letter I have opened it instead.
I love my new bifocals, my dentures fit me fine,
my hearing aid is perfect, but Lord, I miss my mind.

It is easier to extricate oneself from the changes of aging when the changes don't involve one's own personality. While you may be able to see the body as object, it is very hard to see the personality as object because you've identified with it for so long. You think that's who you are. Even though they keep changing, you keep identifying with those thoughts and feelings.

Now we are getting more into the heart of the matter: can you find a place to stand in relation to change where you are not frightened by it? Can you live in the presence of change, even enjoy the changes—work with the changes, become an elder, do all the things that involve changing—and at the same moment cultivate equanimity, clarity, loving awareness, compassion, and joy? Balancing those qualities is really what the deep spiritual work is about.

FREE TO BE

One of the reasons that old age is so disconcerting to many people is that their roles change, and with those changes they experience a loss of purpose; a diminished sense of value, identity, and self-worth; confusion about how to behave; a feeling of no longer being needed. People are uncertain how to restructure their lives, how to manifest as a being whose role is now totally unfamiliar to them. Retirement and having children leave the parental nest are two role changes that come to mind.

Recognize in yourself the conflicting forces; part of you wants to stay effective in the world, and part of you wants to be contemplative. Really give that contemplative part some space. Water it a bit and give it some sunlight to grow instead of treating it as an error. Give yourself the opportunity to grieve—for the end of dreams, for the end of childhood, for all the people that go away, for the sorrow of parting.

When you experience fear or are unsure about your situation, there's a beautiful and very powerful mantra you can say: "The power of God is within me. The grace of God surrounds me." Repeat it to yourself or to a loved one in need. It will protect you. Experience the power of it. It's like a solid steel shaft that goes through the top of your head right down to the base of your being. Grace will surround you like a force field.

One of the gifts of old age is no longer caring so much about what others think of us. Aging allows us to be more eccentric. When we were younger, we were expected to behave in a certain way. As we age, we can let it all fall apart a little more. We are free to be ourselves—to follow our hunches, to experiment, or to do nothing at all—as age liberates us from our old roles and offers a different kind of freedom and an authentic way of being. Nadine Strain was eighty-five when she wrote the poem "If I Had My Life to Live Over":

I'd like to make more mistakes next time. I'd relax. I would limber up.
I would be sillier than I have been this trip. I would take more chances.
I would climb more mountains and swim more rivers.
I would eat more ice cream and less beans.
I would perhaps have more actual troubles, but I'd have fewer
imaginary ones.
You see, I'm one of those people who live sensibly and sanely
*   hour after hour, day after day.*
Oh, I've had my moments, and if I had it to do over again,
I'd have more of them. In fact, I'd try to have nothing else.
Just moments, one after another, instead of living so many years ahead
of each day.
I've been one of those persons who never goes anywhere without a
thermometer, a hot water bottle, a raincoat, and a parachute.
If I had to do it again,
I would travel lighter than I have.
If I had my life to live over, I would start barefoot earlier in the spring
and stay that way later in the fall.
I would go to more dances. I would ride more merry-go-rounds.
I would pick more daisies.

Don't get caught in your old roles. If you cultivate the ways you exist behind personality, the pure awareness of the witness, the "I am loving awareness" place in your heart, you will begin to live more in your soul. If you see the Beloved when you look at another being, then everyone you see is a soul, as well as a mirror for your own soul.

Relationships become so beautiful. Each person's struggle, each person's journey, is so exquisite. Let yourself stop for a moment and appreciate that beauty. It is so precious. Most people have no idea they are beautiful. They're busy being not beautiful, because they think, "If only I had this or that, then I'd be beautiful." But who they are—their pain and their beauty—is all so beautiful.

The Beloved keeps appearing to you in one guise or another. You can cultivate this view and practice your ability to see the soul. Seeing the subtlety inside another person also depends on your ability to acknowledge it in yourself. It takes One to know One.

LETTING GO . . . AGAIN

Conscious aging has to do with letting go, which allows you to come into the present moment—into spirit. Hold on tightly, let go lightly.

Making believe you are done with something you are not truly finished with will slow you down on your journey to God. Equally, trying to hold onto something you are done with will slow your journey.

How do you get on with it? You give up the things that don't get you to God. What do you give up? It's not just material stuff. It's also the ways you identify yourself, how you feel about yourself. For instance, give up your unworthiness. Don't analyze it—just give it up. Keep giving up your guilt, your anger, and your preoccupation with your own melodrama. It's just a melodrama, a soap opera. Don't you already know how it comes out?

You took this birth because you have work to do that involves suffering and the kinds of situations you find yourself in. This is your curriculum for this birth. Where you are now with all your neuroses and problems is just the right place. This is it, and it's perfect. Live life fully and richly as a partner with God and accept what comes with openness and love.

BEING WITH WHAT IS

Expand your perception of the world to include the horrible beauty of decay. Look at decay and see how beautiful it is in its own way. My dear friend Laura Huxley had a collection of beautiful pharmaceutical jars in her kitchen over the sink. She'd take old beet greens and orange peels and things and put them in water in the jars and let them slowly mold and decay into beautiful formations catching the light. It was decay as art. There is true beauty in that.

There's horror and beauty in everything. I look at my hand, and it's decaying. It's beautiful and horrible at the same moment, and I just live with it. See the beauty and perfection of decay in the world around you and in yourself, and just allow it to be.

There are some unappreciated advantages to aging. The very frailty of age guards its secrets. To many people you become irrelevant, which gives you more time to do inner work. Francis, a resident in a nursing home, wrote to me, "Lack of physical strength keeps me inactive and often silent. They call me senile. Senility is a convenient peg on which to hang nonconformity. A new set of faculties seems to be coming into operation. I seem to be waking to a larger world of wonderment—to catch little glimpses of the immensity and diversity of creation. More than at any other time of my life, I seem to be aware of the beauties of our spinning planet and the sky above. Old age is sharpening my awareness."

It is interesting to see how aging can work to one's advantage spiritually. I used to go to Burma to sit in meditation. I'd go into a cell. I'd sit down—no books, no television, no computers, no one to talk to. I'd just sit and go inward. I'd go into as quiet a place as I could find. Just look at what happens when you get old. You lose your hearing, you lose your sight, you can't move around so well, you slow down. What an ideal time to meditate. If any message is clear, that's it. Yet we treat aging as an error or a failing.

That distortion comes from defining ourselves in terms of doing instead of being. But behind all the doing, all the roles, you just *are*—pure awareness, pure consciousness, pure energy. When you reside fully in the present moment, you are outside of time and space.

Trungpa Rinpoche notes, "Our lives awaken through ordinary magic." It's in everyday things that the miraculous happens. If we practice being here now, we develop the sensitivity to perceive and appreciate the daily miracles of our lives.

For a while I lived in an old school bus and spent a lot of time in campgrounds with elderly neighbors. Earlier in their lives these people had focused on planning for the future. Now that the future was here, their consciousness was occupied with the past. I heard heavy doses of sentimental reverie. As I was thinking about this, I wondered, "Whatever happened to the present moment? What happened to just making tea? What happened to this consciousness of just being together in this beautiful place under the stars?"

Their minds were holding onto an identity that they were constantly reinforcing by reliving the past. Any memory of a high moment you've held on to keeps you from this present moment. And right *here* is the living spirit. If not *here*, then nowhere.

Now isn't preparation for later. Here and now is *it*. There is a spaciousness, an acceptance of what is in the moment, that says, "Yes, ah so!" to everything, whether it's ugly, beautiful, boring, confused, dead, angry, the dark night of the soul, or the brilliant light of the spirit. This is just the way it is. And in just the way it is, *is* the spirit.

This moment is just enough. To come more and more fully into the moment is to fully appreciate the infusion of the spirit. Once you've tasted what it's like to be in the spirit, to be with the Beloved, you can't stand to be away. Coming fully into the moment is like coming through a doorway to another dimension of consciousness—into *being here now.*

In *Walden,* Henry David Thoreau wrote:

Sometimes . . . I sat in my sunny doorway from sunrise till noon,
rapt in a reverie, amidst the pines and hickories and sumacs, in the
undisturbed solitude and stillness, while the birds sing around or
flitted noiseless through the house, until by the sun falling in at my
west window, or the noise of some traveller's wagon on the distant

highway, I was reminded of the lapse of time. I grew in those seasons like corn in the night, and they were far better than any work of the hands would have been. They were not time subtracted from my life, but so much over and above my usual allowance. I realized what the Orientals mean by contemplation and the forsaking of works.

In a letter, he also wrote, "To some extent, and at rare intervals, even I am a yogi."

Chapter 5

Conscious Living, Conscious Dying

AGING GIVES US a chance to learn to use the shadows in our life as vehicles for our awakening—and the longest shadow of all is death. How you relate to death is the key spiritual work of aging. And how you see death is a function of how much you identify with that which dies. Egos die. Souls don't die. Rainer Maria Rilke wrote:

> *But this: that one can contain*
> *death, the whole of death,*
> *even before life has begun,*
> *can hold it to one's heart*
> *gently, and not refuse to go on living,*
> *is inexpressible.*

I encourage you to make peace with death, to see it as the culminating event of this adventure called life. Death is not an error; it is not a failure. My astral teacher, Emmanuel, says it is like taking off a tight shoe. Confucius says, "Those that find the Way in the morning can gladly die in the evening."

For some of us, the subject of death is easy to talk about, and for some of us, it's a little threatening and frightening. I recognize all that. But part of the essential spiritual work for us at any age is to find a way to be with death.

An old tombstone inscription reads:

Dear friend,
Please know as you pass by
As you are now, so once was I.
As I am now so you will be.
Prepare yourself to follow me.

Take that epitaph as a blessing from beyond, and let us prepare ourselves. I realize it's presumptuous of me to talk about death, as if I know about it, but I have chutzpah, which is Sanskrit for "a lot of nerve." In my meanderings through realms of consciousness over the past fifty years, something happened to me that changed my attitude toward death. A lot of the fear that surrounds death has left me.

Partly that is from being with my guru and getting glimpses of his perspective. He saw life and death from beyond the physical body, as part of a long parade of births and deaths.

DEALING WITH FEAR

Not everyone is ready to talk with you about dying. We have to honor all of our individual differences. Years ago my father was about to have minor surgery, and the night before, I visited him in the hospital. No operation is minor when you are eighty years old. We had a nice visit. I had my jacket on, and I was halfway out the door when Dad called me back.

"Just in case things go wrong, is there anything I should know?" he asked.

I went back to his bedside and said, "All I can tell you is, as good as this is, that is going to be better. And wherever you go, I'll be there."

Dad said, "Great, that's all I wanted to know. See you later."

For many of us, the thought of death, thinking of when we or someone we love is going to die, keeps us from being here now. When will we die? How will we die? What will happen after we die? What will happen to our loved ones? What about all the things we hoped to accomplish? These deep fears and anxieties about our survival keep us from living fully in the present moment.

Most of us are convinced that we are our egos, which is who we *think* we are. The ego is part of our incarnation. It dies with the body, which is why we are so afraid of death. Death scares the hell out of who you think you are, especially if you think you are this body. Being around death forces you to open to a deeper part of yourself. The shadow, especially the shadow of death, is the greatest teacher for how to come to the light.

That fear of death is an anticipatory fear. The only real preparation for death is the moment-to-moment process of life. When you live in the present moment, you are not living in the future or in the past.

Don't prolong the past,
Don't invite the future,
Don't alter your innate wakefulness,
Don't fear appearances.
There's nothing more than that!
PATRUL RINPOCHE

When you are fully present in the moment, there is no anticipatory fear, no anxiety, because you are just here and now, not in the future. When we are resting in our souls, death is just closing a chapter in a book.

DEALING WITH PAIN

Pain or the fear of pain is one of the major traps for our ego in the process of dying. Although spiritual practices are a great help, pain is a worthy adversary. What helps me the most is identifying with the soul level of consciousness and staying centered in mantra. We are not our bodies, but when our bodies experience pain, that is often difficult to remember. That's one reason it's important to do spiritual practice when we are healthy, so that we remain centered in the spirit when we are not.

Physical pain or emotional pain is a thought as well as a sensation. In working with pain, you witness these thoughts and feelings and don't identify with them. You are not your pain. The pain is in your body and your mind. Try to be present in your soul. It isn't easy; Wavy Gravy sums it up well, "Pain sucks!" Truly relieving the mental and emotional side of pain, your own or anyone else's, depends on maintaining your spiritual center, witnessing from your spiritual heart, and not identifying with the painful sensations, thoughts, and emotions. Pain is a fierce motivator. From the spiritual standpoint, it's one of those places where the rubber meets the road.

In conventional Western medicine, people can now decide for themselves, in collaboration with their doctor, how much pain medication they need. It turns out that when people know that they have control over their pain, they need a lot less medication, because often pain is actually made worse by the fear of pain.

When working with pain, give it space, allow it to be, and know that your awareness of the pain is separate from the pain itself. Opening to the pain allows it to be part of the reality you are witnessing and decreases the resistance to it, allowing you to relax around it. Open to what it is, acknowledge it, give it space, bring your awareness to it as another sensation. Pain is, and you *are*.

Poet and teacher Stephen Levine, in his book *Guided Meditations, Explorations and Healings,* includes a meditation for letting go of pain. He says:

> Consider the possibility that the resistance to the pain and the fear
> pain may evoke may be more painful than the pain itself. Notice
> how the resistance closes your heart and fills your body and mind
> with tension and dis-ease. Keep relaxing the resistance . . . the
> tightness . . . that has accumulated around the pain. "Soften"
> around the pain.

Ginny was a patient at the hospice where I was serving in California. The first time I visited her she was skeptical and asked what I had to teach her. She was dying of cancer of the nervous system, and she was in extreme pain. She said she was bored with dying. I invited her to try being here now, and we did a little practice to bring her into the moment. Outside her open window we could hear children playing. I suggested that she bring the sound of the children inside of her. After a while, I suggested she incorporate the ticking sound of the clock in the room inside of her. She became very present. Coming fully into the moment and into her soul took her out of time and space. This is important in life and even more so when someone is dying. The soul is independent of time and space.

Ginny and I became dear friends. There came a time when she was so weak that all I could do was sit by her bedside. She was literally writhing in pain, twisting her head and rubbing her hands over her body. Her expression was one of very intense pain. I sat next to her, doing the Buddhist meditation on the decaying body. This is a formal meditation on the stages of decay of the human body. I sat there, wide open, not closing my eyes or going off to some other place, just staying with her, noticing the pain, noticing the whole thing. I was letting my emotions flow but not holding on or clinging to them or getting into judgment. I was just watching the laws of the universe unfold, which is not easy to do around death, especially with someone we love, because of our emotional attachment.

As I sat there watching the pain and suffering, I started to experience a great deep calm. The room became luminous. At that moment, though her body was writhing with pain, Ginny turned to me and whispered, "I feel so peaceful." In this meditative environment, she had been able to move beyond the pain and experience deep peace. We had created a vibrational space that we could be in together. Neither she nor I wanted to be in any other place in the universe at that moment. A feeling of bliss permeated the room. All I had done really was not to be freaked out that she was dying or in pain.

WHAT DIES?

Each of us has our own work to do, our own unique karmic predicament. But what's most important is where you are doing it from—that is, your point of view. Are you doing it from your ego, your role, your personality—or from a place in you that doesn't change—your spiritual heart, your soul?

Are you stuck in time or not? Time is a river that flows from birth to death, a lifetime. If you are in time, you will suffer and you will die. If you change your identification from that which dies to your soul, then you move into that realm of awareness that is beyond time, though it includes time. Then you are a soul who is part of the One. And souls don't die.

Rilke said, "Love and death are magnificent gifts, which many of us leave unopened."

Making peace with your feelings about death is the prerequisite for living life joyfully here and now. Death does not have to be treated as an enemy for you to delight in life. Keeping death present in your consciousness as one of the greatest mysteries, as the moment of incredible transformation, imbues *this* moment with added richness and energy.

The minute the fear of death has been faced, the meaning of life changes. Otherwise your fear distorts your perception all the time, and you panic when someone gets near death. That panic is because of your identification with those thoughts.

The journey of consciousness is about arriving at a balance in life where you are open to the mystery of it all. You can't be open when you're loaded down with a lot of conceptual stuff. In my own consciousness, I watch how long it takes, when an expectation isn't fulfilled, before I come back again to being in the present moment. How long before I can let go of not getting what I wanted, and just be with what is?

As long as you identify with the part of you that dies, there is always fear of death, because it is the fear of cessation of existence. Through my experiences with psychedelic mushrooms in the '60s, I had the ineffable, profound experience of pure consciousness beyond my body and knowing that this essence of my awareness is beyond death. It was soon after that Aldous Huxley gave *The Tibetan Book of the Dead* to Tim Leary and me. Lamas read aloud from this book to their fellow monks when they are dying and in the days following death. The book is centuries old, yet described the same experiences I had with the mushrooms, bringing me full circle to the universal nature of these experiences.

These issues of death, pain, and suffering bring us to the very limit of our mind's ability to deal with the mystery of life. Many people rely on religion to reassure them about death. But religious teachings are belief systems that are part of the mind structure, and fear is inherent in a belief system, because when you die, your mind dies and your beliefs die with it. A belief won't keep you warm on a cold night.

What may serve you is faith. Not faith in something outside—I mean living *in* faith. It is faith in the sense that I live in absolute wonder, in the presence of the great mystery.

In our Western culture, although death has come out of the closet, it is still not openly experienced or discussed. Living in India, I found the differences in our outlook on death and theirs to be enormous. In India, death is a familiar part of life. Allowing dying to be so intensely present enriches both the preciousness of each moment and our detachment from it.

In India it is not unusual to see a body being carried down the street on the way to the burning *ghat* to be cremated. The body leaves with the head facing back to its physical home. Halfway to the burning ghat, the body is turned around, so the head is facing the opposite direction, toward the burning ghat, to symbolize the transition to the spiritual home. The whole way, people in the procession are chanting, "Rām Nām Sathya Hai, Sathya Bol, Sathya Hai," which means, "Rām's [God's] name is Truth."

One day Maharaj-ji was walking with a devotee of many years when he suddenly looked up and said, "Ma just died." She was an old woman and a great devotee. Since she lived in a distant city, it was obvious he had seen her death on another plane. Then he laughed and laughed. His devotee was shocked and called Maharaj-ji a "butcher" to laugh at the death of such a beautiful and pure woman. Maharaj-ji turned and said, "What do you want me to do, act like one of the puppets?"

Maharaj-ji often spoke about death to his devotees, and his perceptions had a major effect on my attitude about dying. Some of the things he said were, "The body passes away. Everything is impermanent except the love of God," and, "The body dies, but not the soul." He also said, "This world is all attachment. Yet you get worried because you are attached."

When the great South Indian saint Ramana Maharshi was dying of cancer, his doctors wanted to treat him, but he refused, saying, "This body is all used up." His devotees, who loved him dearly, cried, "Bhagawan [Blessed One], don't leave us, don't leave us." He replied, "Don't be silly, where can I go?"

The biblical idea of dying and the soul being born again into truth or wisdom or spirit is what our business with death is really about. As the Bhagavad Gita says, "We are born into the world of nature; our second birth is into the world of spirit."

As you extricate yourself from a rigid identification with body, personality, and mind, you begin to be spacious enough to allow death to be part of the process of life rather than the end of existence. I feel this very deeply.

People ask me if I believe there is continuity after death. I say that I don't believe it—it just is. This offends my scientific friends no end. But belief is something you hold with your intellect, and for me this goes way beyond my intellect. The Bhagavad Gita also tells us, "As the Spirit of our mortal body wanders on in childhood and youth and old age, the Spirit wanders on to a new body: of this the sage has no doubts." As Krishna says, "Because we all have been for all time . . . And we all shall be for all time, we all for ever and ever."

In a Buddhist country in an ancient time, an army was going through villages and killing many people. They were disemboweling the monks to get rid of Buddhism, which happened a lot in the times of Genghis Khan. There was one particularly harsh commander who had a reputation for being very cruel. He came into this town, and he said to his adjutant, "What's happening in the town?"

The adjutant said, "All the people are bowing down to you. They are all afraid of you. All the monks in the monastery have fled to the mountains except for one monk."

The commander was furious that a monk was still there. He walked into the monastery and pushed open the gates, and there in the middle of the courtyard was the monk just standing there. The captain walked up to him and said, "Don't you know who I am? I could take my sword and run it through your belly without blinking an eye."

"And don't you know who I am?" said the monk, "I could have your sword run through my belly without blinking an eye."

The commander bowed and left.

When you get into the spiritual literature, you start to see a lightness about death. A Zen master was dying. Zen masters are supposed to leave a death verse, and he hadn't written his yet. His students were very concerned that he would die before writing his verse. They kept saying, "What about your verse? What about your verse?" So he picked up his calligraphy brush and wrote, "Earth is thus, death is thus. Verse or no verse, what's the fuss?" And then he died.

In his foreword to a 1960 edition of *The Tibetan Book of the Dead*, Lama Anagarika Govinda wrote:

> It may be argued that nobody can talk about death with authority who has not died; and since nobody, apparently, has ever returned from death, how does anybody know what death is, or what happens after it?
>
> The Tibetan will answer: "There is not *one* person, indeed, not *one* living being, that has *not* returned from death. In fact, we have all died many deaths before we came into this incarnation. And what we call birth is merely the reverse side of death," like one of the two sides of a coin, or like a door which we call "entrance" from outside and "exit" from inside a room.
>
> It's much more astonishing that not everybody remembers his or her previous death; and, because of this lack of remembering, most persons do not believe there was a previous death. But, likewise, they do not remember their birth—and yet they do not doubt that they were recently born.

BEING WITH SOMEONE DYING

I sit with people who are dying. I'm one of those unusual types that enjoys being with someone when they're dying because I know I am going to be in the presence of Truth. I was with my mother and later my stepmother when they were dying. I am deeply grateful for those experiences.

My mother was dying in early February, 1966, in a hospital in Boston. I was sitting at her bedside. By then I had been working on understanding my own consciousness for some years. She was sort of resting. I was in kind of a meditative mode, just being spacious and aware and noticing what was happening as the relatives and doctors and nurses came into the hospital room and said, "Gertrude, how are you doing?" I listened to the cheery tone of the nurse. I realized that my mother was surrounded by a conspiracy of denial. I watched people coming into the room, all the relatives and doctors and nurses saying she was looking better, that she was doing well, and then they would go out of the room and say she wouldn't live out the week. I thought how bizarre it was that a human being going through one of the most profound transitions in her life was completely surrounded by deception. Can you hear the pain of that? One woman came in and said, "The doctor just told me there's a new medication that we think will help."

Nobody could be straight with her because everybody was too frightened—all of them, everybody, even the rabbi. Mother and I talked about it. At one point, when nobody else was in the room, she turned to me and said, "Rich?" I'd just been sitting there—no judgment, no nothing, just sitting—and we just met in that space.

She said, "Rich, I think I'm going to die."

I said, "Yeah, I think so too."

Imagine what that must have been for her to just have somebody affirm what she knew. She couldn't get anybody in the entire constellation of her friends, relatives, doctors, and nurses to validate it for her.

She said, "What do you think it's going to be like, Rich?"

I said, "Well, of course, I don't know. But I look at you, and I can see your body disintegrating. It's like a house burning. But you are still there, and I figure when the building burns, it will go, and you'll still be there. It seems to me the way you and I are connected isn't really defined by this body that is disintegrating, because you sound just like you've always sounded. I feel like I've always felt. Yet this body is decaying before us.

"I think the way that you and I love each other, I just believe that love transcends death." That was a very touching connection for us.

Later I was with my stepmother, Phyllis, when she was dying of cancer. Phyllis was sixty-nine, and my father was eighteen years older. When they got married, I gave away the bride. We were good buddies. Now she was dying, and my role was to be with her and help her through the process.

She and I had been to the doctors together, and we had done the whole thing of getting all the reports and dealing with all the emotions. Phyllis was a very tough New England lady, a wonderful, grounded, poker-playing woman. She was argumentative and willful, just fun.

She had a stiff-upper-lip way of living life, and she was approaching her death the same way. My job wasn't to say, "Hey, Phyllis, you should open to this." That wasn't my moral right. My job was just to be there with her. So I would lie on the bed, and we would hold each other, and we would just talk. We would talk about death and what we thought it might be like and all, but she was still being very strong.

The pain of the cancer was intense, and over time it finally wore away her will. A moment came, maybe four or five days before her death, when she gave up.

In our culture giving up is seen as a failure. Everybody says to keep trying, keep trying. The result is we sometimes surround dying people with a kind of false hope that comes out of our own fear.

With Phyllis, I was just open, and she could ask whatever she wanted. I didn't say, "Now let me instruct you about dying," because she wouldn't have accepted that. But then she gave up. At the moment she surrendered, it was like watching an egg hatch. A new being emerged that was so radiantly beautiful and present and light and joyful. It was a being that at some deep intuitive level she knew herself to be but never had time for in her adult life. She opened to this being, and together we just basked in its radiance. At that moment she had gone into another plane of consciousness. We were together talking, but the pain and the dying process had just become phenomena. She was no longer busy dying; she was just being, and dying was happening.

Just to complete this story, to tell you how extraordinary this transformation was, right at the last moment she said, "Richard, please sit me up."

So I sat her up. I put her legs over the bed, and her body was falling forward. So I put my hand on her chest, and her body fell back. So I put my other hand on her back, and her head was lolling. So I put my head against her head. We were just sitting there together. She took three breaths—slow, deep breaths—and she left.

If you read the ancient Tibetan texts, you read that when conscious lamas leave their body, they sit up, they take three breaths, and they leave. Who was Phyllis? How did she know that? What was that about? These are the mysteries that we live with.

My dear friend Deborah was dying at Memorial Hospital in New York. She was a member of the New York Zen Center, and every evening her friends from the center came to her hospital room to meditate. Doctors entering this hospital room were surprised to find it lit by candles and filled with the fragrance of incense and the deep peace of people in meditation. In this busy big-city hospital, this group of people meditating had redefined the metaphor for dying. You can create your universe anywhere you are. A hospital is merely a collective of beings who share a certain model about what it's all about. Each night her doctors entered the room more gently.

Curing a disease of the body is not always an option, but healing from the soul level is always possible. In working with those who are dying, I offer another human being a spacious environment with my mind in which they can die as they need to die. I have no right to define how another person should die. I'm just there to help them transition, however they need to do it. My role is just to be a loving rock at the bedside.

When Wavy Gravy, the clown prince of the Hog Farm commune, talks to children about dying, he tells them to shed their body like taking off a suit of old clothes and to go for the light that will take you to God, your friend.

Working with the dying is like being a midwife for this great rite of passage of death. Just as a midwife helps a being take their first breath, you help a being take their last breath. To be there fully requires being deeply grounded in compassion and love. Compassion, in this instance, is just both of you becoming who you are together—like the right hand taking care of the left hand.

In *Guided Meditations, Explorations and Healings,* Stephen Levine says:

Death is an illusion we all seem to buy into. . . . But death, like anything that catches the heart's attention, can bring out the best in us. We have seen many people as they approach even the confusion around death, go beyond that dismay and become one with the process. . . . They deepen the work they perhaps took birth to complete. They are no longer someone separate, someone "dying consciously." They are merely space within space, light within light.

See in the dying person only that which is eternal. Then you will be able to communicate as souls.

When you are with someone who is dying, *be there* with them. All you have to give is your own being. Be honest. Meditate and become aware that the pain or confusion *is,* and here we are, in quiet equanimity. We all have limits of tolerance. Stay as clear and conscious as possible as someone nears death. Open to the unexpected. Open and stay centered. If you remain centered, your calm presence helps to free all those around you. Go inside yourself to that quiet place where you *are* wisdom. Wisdom has in it compassion. Compassion understands about life and death. The answer to dying is to be present in the moment. To learn to die is to learn how to live. And the way you do that is by living each moment—this one, now this one—just being here now.

The moment when the soul leaves the body is palpable and deeply profound. To share consciousness with a person who is dying, to be with them and help them die consciously, is one of the most exquisite manifestations of service. It is one role you may want to try out.

CONSCIOUS DYING

My view has evolved to seeing death—the moment of death—as a ceremony. If people are sitting with you to help as you are going through this dying ceremony, help them to see you as the soul you truly are, not as your ego. If they identify you as your ego, during the last part of this ceremony they will cling to you and pull you back instead of facilitating your transformation.

Sadhana, either a specific practice or your overall spiritual transformation, begins with you as an ego and evolves into your being a soul, who you really are. The ego is identified with the incarnation, which stops at the moment of death. The soul, on the other hand, has experienced many deaths. If you've done your sadhana fully, there will be no fear of death, and dying is just another moment.

If you are to die consciously, there's no time like the present to prepare. Here is a brief checklist of some of the ways to approach your own death:

- Live your life consciously and fully. Learn to identify with and be present in your soul, not your ego.
- Fill your heart with love. Turn your mind toward God, guru, Truth.
- Continue with all of your spiritual practices: meditation, mantra, kirtan, all forms of devotion.
- Be there for the death of your parents, loved ones, or beloved animals. Know that the presence of your loved ones will remain when you are quiet and bring them into your consciousness.
- Read about the deaths of great saints, lamas, and yogis like Ramana Maharshi.
- If there is pain at the time of death, try to remain as conscious as possible. Medication for pain offers some solace but dulls your awareness.
- To be peaceful at the time of your death, seek peace inside today. Death is another moment. If you're not peaceful today, you probably won't be peaceful tomorrow.

Sudden death is, in many ways, more difficult to work with spiritually than a gradual passing. If we are aware that death can happen at any moment, we start to work on ourselves more constantly, paying attention to the moment-to-moment content of our minds. If you practice being here now, being fully in the moment during your life, if you are living in that space, then the moment of death is just another moment. Let me tell you a story about living like this.

A monk is being chased by a tiger. He runs as fast as he can, but the tiger is hot on his heels. Ahead of him is a cliff, with a vine hanging down over the edge. He grasps the vine and begins to clamber down the face of the mountain, when down below, he spots another tiger prowling on a ledge beneath him. A tiger above and a tiger below, he hangs there, clinging to the vine. Then he notices that two little mice have scampered up and begun gnawing at the vine that is supporting him. At that desperate moment, he sees right before him a ripe, red, wild strawberry, growing on the side of the mountain. He plucks and eats it—how sweet it tastes!

In Tibet, when they give instructions at the end of life, they say, "As the earth element leaves, your body will feel heavy. As the water element leaves, you will feel dryness. As the fire element leaves, you may feel cold. As the air element leaves, your out-breath will be longer than your in-breath. The signs are now here. Don't get lost in the details. Let your awareness go free." Imagine that, instead of, "Oh I'm thirsty," or "She's thirsty. Give her water," an acknowledgment of, "Ah, the water element."

A feeling of expansion as you go into death—that's just one metaphor. Our concept of going from one plane to another is like climbing rungs on a ladder, or as we said earlier, tuning to another channel on the TV. You have to let go when you leave the physical plane. When I was guiding psychedelic trips, people would bad-trip because they couldn't let go as their consciousness expanded and they faced eternity. You have to let go of your individuality, your name, your history, your friends, your cat, your body. That letting go is meeting the infinite.

Empty your mind of all thoughts.
Let your heart be at peace. . . .
Each separate being in the universe
returns to the common source.
Returning to the source is serenity.
If you don't realize the source,
you stumble in confusion and sorrow.
When you realize where you come from,

you naturally become tolerant,
disinterested, amused,
kindhearted as a grandmother,
dignified as a king.
Immersed in the wonder of the Tao,
you can deal with whatever life brings you,
and when death comes, you are ready.
LAO-TZU, TRANSLATED BY STEPHEN MITCHELL

Whatever you need to do to get ready to die, you should have done it a minute ago. Do it now and get ready. Every moment is the moment you die. Every breath is the first and last. A conscious being holds on nowhere.

GRIEVING

I often work with family members who have lost someone and are grieving. They are grieving for their connection to the place in themselves where they feel safe in the universe and at home, loved, and at peace. When someone close dies, that feeling of safety and security is overturned. I encourage people to stay with what they are feeling—with their grief.

Our Western culture says, "It's good that you're over it. Now you can start living life again." But our attachments to our loved ones are very deep, and grieving has to run its course. Just allow that pain of being human. The passage of time is healing. During this healing phase, surround and insulate yourself with love.

You will grieve and go through all the emotional responses. Then there will come a moment when all of a sudden, you awaken to the fact that the love that you shared with that person is still here. Maybe you will be watching a sunset or just sitting quietly. At that moment you will begin to let go of that person as a separate entity, and allow them to merge into your soul . . . in love.

When you and another person enter into love together, you enter into a unitive moment that transcends death. Recognize that you feel enriched by everybody you have loved, instead of deprived by the loss of their form. You'll realize they continue to live in your heart. Everybody you have ever loved is part of the fabric of your being. And that is where grief gets transformed into a living, loving space, a spiritual transcendence of the pain.

Love transcends death. Still, to *be* that wisdom is different than knowing about it. Death is only a moment, a moment of transition. If you know yourself to be your soul, you've gone through many, many deaths of your own—through many different incarnations. Those whom you are grieving for are also souls passing through deaths, births, deaths, births.

If you identify with your own soul, you will be able to communicate with other souls, even though they are on a different plane. I still communicate with my guru, although he died in 1973. After he died, he was everywhere.

Eleven-year-old Rachael and her girlfriend went to a neighborhood Jewish community center to play tennis, and Rachael was raped and murdered. I received a call that night from a friend who told me the parents had read my books and listened to my tapes.

Was there something I could say to them at this moment? I realized I couldn't do it tomorrow. It had to be done right now because the enormity of that pain was so great. So I wrote this letter to them that I would like to share with you:

Dear Steve and Anita,

Rachael finished her work on Earth and left the stage in a manner that leaves those of us left behind with a cry of agony in our hearts as the fragile thread of our faith is dealt with so violently. Is anyone strong enough to stay conscious through such teachings as you are receiving? Very few, and even they would have only the briefest whisper of equanimity and peace amidst the screaming trumpets of their rage, grief, horror, and desolation.

I can't assuage your pain with any words, nor should I, for your pain is part of Rachael's legacy to you. Not that she or I would inflict such pain by choice, but there it is. And it must burn its purifying way to completion. For something in you dies when you bear the unbearable, and it is only in that dark night of the soul that you are prepared to see as God sees and to love as God loves.

Now is the time to let your grief find expression. No false strength. Now is the time to sit quietly and speak to Rachael and thank her for being with you these few years and encourage her to go on with her work, knowing that you will grow in compassion and wisdom from this experience.

In my heart I know that you and she will meet again and again and recognize the many ways in which you have known each other. And when you meet, you will, in a flash, know what now is not given to you to know and why this had to be the way it was. Our rational minds can never understand what has happened, but our hearts, if we can keep them open to God, will find their own intuitive way.

Rachael came through you to do her work on earth, which included her manner of death. Now her soul is free, and the love that you can share with her is invulnerable to the winds of changing time.

Love,

Ram Dass

DEATH IS A REMINDER TO LIVE LIFE FULLY

In Eastern traditions, the state of consciousness at the last moment of life is considered so crucial that you spend your whole life preparing for it. Mahatma Gandhi, the great Indian leader, walked into a garden to give a press conference and was assassinated. As he fell, all he said was "Rām!" the name of God.

Meher Baba proclaimed, "The divine Beloved is always with you, in you, and around you. Know that you are not separate from Him."

I am without form, without limit
Beyond space, beyond time
I am in everything, everything is in me
I am the bliss of the Universe
Everything Am I
SWAMI RAM TIRTHA

Aldous Huxley says so beautifully in his novel *Island,* "So now you can let go, my darling. . . . Let go. . . . Let go of this poor old body. You don't need it anymore. Let it fall away from you. Leave it lying there like a pile of worn-out clothes. . . . Go on, my darling, go on into the Light, into the peace, into the living peace of the Clear Light."

Making peace with death and being fully in the moment allows you to lose yourself in love—in the love of the beauty and awe of God made manifest, in loving yourself and everything else, the suffering, the pain, the joy. In the eternal present of the moment you are free of time. Then if death is the moment, that's the moment. When you are in that place of openness, it's all possible. At the moment of death, you are surrendering and being cradled in the arms of God. If we let go lightly, we go out into the Light, toward the One, toward God. What grace!

One dies as one lives. What else can better prepare you to die than the way you live? The game is to be where you are—honestly, consciously, and as fully as you know how. Once you have awakened, you can't fully go back to sleep. Regardless of what happens in the world, I'm still going to follow Maharaj-ji's instructions every day—to love everyone, serve everyone, and remember God—love, serve, remember.

There comes a point where you really want to clean up your act. You start to look for the fire of purification. That's when it gets very interesting, because suddenly you're looking for those situations that push your buttons. You take a deeper look at the roles you play in your incarnation—your responsibilities to parents, children, country, religion, friends, yourself—and work on bringing them into harmony with your deeper being.

Part of your relationship with yourself is taking responsibility for the care of your body and doing the things that promote good health. The body is the temple of the soul, the temple of your spirit. It is the vehicle for you to stay in this incarnation and become a fully conscious being—the vehicle for you to become one with God. Honor it. Take care of it. I was not fully conscious in the way I dealt with my body, and I paid a big price with the stroke that I had.

As you quiet your mind, you begin to see the different components of your being and which ones are out of harmony. For example, at times you can feel that your body is pulling on you. It's draining your energy, or the muscles need strengthening or relaxing. Remembering that your body is the temple of your spirit, work with it, doing things that release or balance energy. Hatha yoga, the yoga of energy, can be used as a path to the soul. Forming an asana is talking to God. Also be mindful of what you put into your body. The human body is a manifestation of God. Honor it.

Much of spiritual work is slowing down enough to let our minds come into harmony with our hearts. In the Bhagavad Gita, Krishna tells Arjuna, "Give Me your mind and your heart and you will come to Me." It is as if he is saying, "Always think of me, always love me, and I will guide your heart and your actions." If, as I do, you follow the path of guru kripa, the grace of the guru, the same applies. Let your love and devotion guide the heart. Let the thinking mind be balanced by the bhakti heart.

Being here now is experiential. When you are in the moment, time slows down. In this moment you have all the time in the world. But don't waste a moment. Who you really are is beyond time. When Christ says, "Look, I am making all things new," it's the same as when you're living in the here and now and you start fresh in every new moment. When you are really in this moment, this is all there is. And the moment of death is just another moment.

Chapter 6

From Suffering to Grace

THERE ARE TIMES when each of us has to bear the unbearable. It may come as physical pain, illness, or emotional suffering of our own, of someone dear to us, or of other sentient beings.

Can you respond to suffering without closing down and still keep your heart open? It seems almost instinctive to use your mind to protect your heart, to rationalize the suffering to avoid the pain or discomfort. But then you cut yourself off from true compassion for yourself and others.

Most of us armor our hearts when dealing with the immensity of the suffering that exists in the world. We look at all the people who are starving when we have just finished a big breakfast, and we turn away. We feel like there is nothing we can do, and we can't bear to see the suffering. Armoring the heart is the opposite of opening the heart. You know the feeling of loving another person; you know how that love feeds you. Love is how we feed each other, but when you experience overwhelming suffering, you close your heart defensively. Your heart may feel protected and less vulnerable, but it is also deadened in the process. Armoring the heart cuts off the living spiritual interchange of energy that exists in the universe and that nourishes the spirit in all of us.

We all fear suffering. People find the world scary because they become overwhelmed by the suffering around them, their own and everybody else's. In any major city in the United States, there are homeless people sleeping in doorways. It's one thing to experience this in India; in Calcutta it seems like half the population lives on the street. But in the affluent United States, it's bizarre that some people live so well and some are so poor. It feels like we should be able to get it together enough to provide everybody with at least shelter, food, and clothing. Are we turning away because our minds are closing off our hearts to the suffering of others?

I deal with the immensity of the suffering all around me by cultivating more than one plane of consciousness, by witnessing, and by acknowledging the laws of the universe. When I can arrive at a perceptual vantage point where I look at a leaf or a drop of water or stars and planets and see the oneness of existence, I can begin to see the exquisite interrelationship of phenomena. I can find universal law in each field I examine—physics, astronomy, music, genetics, mathematics, chemistry. From that point of view of oneness, I can't help being filled with awe at the magnificence of how it all works. I also realize that suffering is part of the way it all works.

WHY IS THERE SUFFERING?

After the Buddha's enlightenment under the Bodhi tree, he expounded to his new disciples what came to be known as the Four Noble Truths. The first Noble Truth says that all existence is characterized by suffering. Birth has in it suffering, death has in it suffering, old age has in it suffering, and sickness has in it suffering. Not getting what you want has in it suffering; getting what you don't want has in it suffering. Even getting what you do want or not getting what you don't want involves suffering, because both are in time.

Anything in time is impermanent. Jesus said, "Lay not up for yourselves treasures upon earth, where moth and rust doth corrupt." As long as you are caught up in time, there is suffering. The second and third Noble Truths deal with the causes of suffering, which are the clinging of mind—to attractions and aversions—and to a false sense of self. The fourth Noble Truth lays out the Eightfold Path to get free of suffering.

THE WAY OF GRACE

I deeply honor the Buddha, and I have studied Buddhism a lot and practiced much Buddhist meditation. But my particular spiritual path is through my guru, Maharaj-ji. The guru reflects our deepest Self. Indeed, when fully known, the guru is our deepest Self, and that is who we see when we polish the mirror of our being.

My relationship with Maharaj-ji is one of faith. That faith allows me to see everything that comes my way as his grace. Just remembering that everything is his grace, is itself grace, but sometimes it doesn't come easy.

On February 19, 1997, I suffered a severe hemorrhagic stroke (a bleed rather than a blockage). I had been working on a book about aging, and I was lying in bed trying to imagine what it would be like to be old and sick and suffering, when I had a massive stroke.

The phone rang. I tried to get out of bed to answer it, and I fell onto the floor. I was paralyzed on one side. I managed to reach the phone and pick up the receiver, but I was unable to speak. My friend calling from New Mexico realized something was wrong, and asked me to tap on the phone if I needed help, which I did.

Within a few minutes, my secretaries, Marlene and JoAnne, appeared, soon followed by paramedics. I remember being wheeled into the hospital on a gurney. During those first few days, no one knew if I would survive. The news of my stroke traveled fast—even to India. Prayer circles around the country were sending me healing energy. The people surrounding me, the doctors and nurses, my friends and relatives—all wore long faces. They kept saying, "Oh, you poor guy, you've had a stroke!"

As I absorbed their mindsets, I started to think I was a poor guy, just another stroke victim. They were projecting the full view of a stroke as a medical disaster onto me. It was coming from almost everybody—except the cleaning woman. Whenever she came into my room, she was totally present with me. She *knew*.

Before my stroke, I felt like I led a life of grace because I was under the protective umbrella of my guru. The stroke shattered my faith in that protection. I felt I had fallen out of grace. I lost faith and I got very depressed for a while.

I would look at the picture of my guru on the hospital wall and say, "Where were you when I had this stroke? Were you out to lunch?" For the first two months, I was almost totally dependent and suffering—physically, psychologically, and spiritually. I sat in my hospital bed attempting to make sense of what had happened. On one hand, there was the stroke; on the other hand, there was Maharaj-ji's grace. How did this stroke fit in with his grace?

Slowly things began to shift. I started thinking about the stroke in different ways. Could this stroke be grace in any way? Awful grace? It certainly wasn't helping my ego, but could it possibly benefit my soul? The effects of the stroke included aphasia, paralysis, and dependence on others. Attempting to reperceive it, I tried to find out where the grace might be hidden. After all, this was still Maharaj-ji's play, his *lila*. I was trying to figure out Maharaj-ji's grace in the stroke, how this sickness was going to help get me to God.

Early on I was markedly aphasic, unable to speak at all. Learning to speak again was hard. Words came slowly. I had to learn to deal with silence—a great boon spiritually because it forced my mind to be quiet. I had to go beyond my intellect into the silence of my intuitive heart. As I became more absorbed in the heart, I found it to be a place where separation disappears and knowledge gives way to wisdom. About a year and a half after my stroke, I started speaking again publicly. It's good motivation for your speech therapy to have five hundred people waiting for you to get your words out.

When I would lecture before the stroke, there would always be one or two people in the audience who had been dragged to hear me speak by a spouse or a friend. It was easy to pick them out of the crowd; they'd be sitting with their arms folded and their faces wearing a long-suffering look. I'd work hard to help them open their hearts. Now my wheelchair opened their hearts. And because of the wheelchair, I was always assured of having a seat wherever I went.

The stroke taught me about dependency. I went from being the driver of a sports car to a passenger. I was in a body that now needed help from others. As a passenger I could appreciate the passing trees and clouds in a way I couldn't when I had to pay attention to traffic.

I had written a book called *How Can I Help?* (with Paul Gorman); now I needed to write one called, *How Can You Help Me?* Since the stroke, I have been deeply humbled by the compassion of other beings. I am blessed to have such wonderful people taking care of me. Now they take care of my body, and together we take care of each other's souls.

CHANGING YOUR POINT OF VIEW

As I see it, we have three vantage points, or planes of consciousness, from which we live. The first is the ego, the plane of personality. The second is our individual soul, part of which is the witness consciousness we talked about earlier. The third is the mystic part of us. Quakers call it the still, small voice within, or the inner light. Hindus call it the Atmān. We can also think of it as the One.

Each of us has all three of these channels. They are all here simultaneously, but how you experience reality depends on which one your awareness is tuned to. When you dwell deep in the intuitive self, you are on the soul plane. If you follow that awareness and go in and in, you will come to God awareness, to the Atmān. That same awareness is in you and in me. God consciousness is the same in all of us. While we think we are our incarnation, our soul witnesses it all, and ultimately connects us to the universal God consciousness that dwells within each of us.

These days I see myself as a soul who has taken incarnation in a body that suffered a stroke. So while my ego thought I was a person with a stroke, that suffering pushed me into my soul, which witnesses or watches the incarnation. It's much less painful to watch the stroke than to have the stroke.

I have pains throughout my body. I list them for my doctors. But I don't identify with them. I identify with being a witness of pain. Physical pain is in the body, and I am not my body. My body is out there, and I am in here. Pain is part of the body. Now if we're talking about psychological pain, that is from the ego, which is also out there. I remember I am my consciousness, my awareness. I am inside, and I live with the pain—not *as* the pain, but *with* the pain.

That is another way the stroke proved beneficial: it pushed me into my soul. Instead of leaving me wallowing in the physical problems of my incarnation, it gave me a leg up and took me into my soulness.

IS IT SUFFERING OR IS IT GRACE?

Recall the story from the *Rāmayana* in which Ravana, the demon king, kidnaps Sita, the earth mother or the soul who is married to God, Rām. He carries her away to the demon capital on the island of Sri Lanka. As the army of monkeys and bears arrives at the ocean shore in India looking for Sita, Jambavan, the king of the bears, reminds Hanuman that he has divine powers. Then Hanuman takes his great leap of faith and flies over the ocean to find Sita.

As I struggled in my mind to accept this stroke, a message came from a dear friend in India. In the same way that Hanuman needed to be reminded of his power, my friend K.K. Sah in India felt I should be reminded of the power of my faith. K.K. wrote some simple words that Maharaj-ji had said to him about me: "I will do something for him." Just that remembrance was enough to recall my faith. My soul was once again enveloped in Maharaj-ji's blanket of love.

Siddhi Ma, the "Mother" in India who maintains Maharaj-ji's ashrams, saw Mickey Lemle's documentary film about me and the stroke, which was called *Fierce Grace*. In the film, I talked about trying to see the stroke as Maharaj-ji's grace. She sent me a message that Maharaj-ji would never give me a stroke. I finally realized that the stroke was the natural result of my own karma. Maharaj-ji's grace lay in helping me deal with the effects of the stroke. It is true that being able to deal with the suffering from the stroke changed my life.

I certainly wouldn't wish a stroke on anyone, but mine has had its positive side. Although I lost my faith for a while, over time it has been tempered and deepened. Although for a time I was overwhelmed by the suffering, eventually I found a place in myself that has faith that this stroke is part of my awakening. That was the grace.

Living with both the perfection and the pain of the suffering allows me to stay with the pain without pushing it away, because I have that balance within myself. I'm part of the unfolding of it all, and that includes suffering.

When Phyllis, my stepmother, was dying, the pain she went through forced her to give up clinging to her body and led to her spiritual awakening during the few days before she died. I wouldn't have given her that pain, but who am I to judge? As a human being with an emotional heart, I am faced with the paradox that I want to relieve suffering, while at the same moment there is another part of me that understands that sometimes there is grace in suffering. From a spiritual point of view, suffering is sometimes the sandpaper that awakens people. Once you start to awaken spiritually, you reperceive your own suffering and start to work with it as a vehicle for further awakening.

When you suffer, the suffering seems to envelop your world. Think of a framed picture of a cloud. If the picture is cropped too closely, you see only the gray of the cloud. If the picture is cropped to a wider angle, you see the blue sky all around it. That's grace.

FAITH

The whole game is based on faith. Faith comes through grace. In the Bible, the apostle Paul says, "For it is by grace you have been saved, through faith—and this is not from yourselves, it is the gift of God—not by works, so that no one can boast."

When the faith is strong enough, it is sufficient just to be. Without faith, the existential fears and uncertainties that we all have dominate. If you have faith, you have no fear. If you don't have faith, you fear.

As I questioned my own faith after the stroke, I began to ask, "Faith in what?" I found that my faith is in the One—not faith in Maharaj-ji as a person, but faith in him as a doorway to the One, faith in the One in Maharaj-ji. Oneness is a state of being. Again, this is the state where, as the great South Indian saint Ramana Maharshi said, "God, guru, and Self are one." Maharaj-ji simply held up one finger and said, "Sub ek"—it's all One.

Faith is the reflection of that oneness in the mirror of your soul. Faith is the way you connect to that universal truth of oneness. Faith and love are intimately entwined. As it says in the *Rāmayana,* without devotion, there is no faith; without faith, there is no devotion.

Faith is not a belief. Beliefs are in the head. Faith is in the heart. Faith comes from within you. You cultivate it by opening your spiritual heart and quieting your mind until you feel your identity with your deeper Self. That opening to the deeper Self, when you have quieted your mind. comes through grace. The qualities of that Self are peace, joy, compassion, wisdom, and love.

IT'S ALL PERFECT

Having been in the presence of Maharaj-ji, I have come to trust the way a being like that is in the universe. It's like knowing somebody who lives a little farther up the mountain and can see farther than you can. The view from there is perfection—not perfection as something to be achieved, but perfection in what is. Maharaj-ji kept saying to me in various ways, "Ram Dass, don't you see it's all perfect?" And yet Maharaj-ji spent all his life being there for people, helping them with their lives, feeding them, and just loving them.

The art of life is to stay wide open and be vulnerable, yet at the same time to sit with the mystery and the awe and with the unbearable pain—to just be with it all. I've been growing into that wonderful catchphrase, "be here now," for the last forty years. Here and now has within it a great richness that is just enough.

If somebody asks me, "Ram Dass, are you happy?" I stop and look inside. "Yes, I'm happy." "Ram Dass, are you sad?" "Yes, I'm sad." Answering those questions, I realize that all of those feelings are present. Imagine the richness of a moment in which everything is present: the pain of a broken heart, the joy of a new mother holding her baby, the exquisiteness of a rose in bloom, the grief of losing a loved one. This moment has all of that. It is just living truth.

The saving grace is being able to witness suffering from the perspective of the soul. Another way to say it is that the saving grace is having faith. Living in the fullness of the moment with joy and suffering, witnessing it in all its perfection, our hearts still go out to those who are suffering.

If we live in the moment, we are not in time. If you think, "I'm a retired person. I've retired from my role," you are looking back at your life. It's retrospective; it's life in the rearview mirror. If you're young, you might be thinking, "I have my whole life ahead of me. This is what I'll do later." That kind of thinking is called time binding. It causes us to focus on the past or the future and to worry about what comes next.

Getting caught up in memories of the past or worrying about the future is a form of self-imposed suffering. Either retirement or youth can be seen as moving on, a time for something different, something new. Start fresh. It's a new moment. Aging is not a culmination. Youth isn't preparation for later. This isn't the end of the line or the beginning. Now isn't a time to look back or plan ahead. It's time to just be present. The present is timeless. Being in the moment, just being here with what is, is ageless, eternal.

It is extraordinary how near we are to our deeper being. It's just a thought away. And the thoughts that take us away from it create so much suffering. The thought "I am this body" causes suffering. I might think, "Well, my body used to be able to do this. My hair didn't used to be gray. I used to be stronger. I used to be thinner. I used to be . . ." Those thoughts cause suffering because the body is what it is. We do everything we can to stay safe and healthy, but illness, age, and accidents still affect us. Maharaj-ji said, "No one has the power even to keep their own body safe." The Buddha is right: this body is in time. But we are just here, in this moment.

GIVING CARING

If you have had the grace to touch living spirit in your lifetime, you know it can be a challenge to translate it into action in the world. To put it another way, now that you know that home is where the heart is, how do you live your life in such a way as to deepen your spiritual connection? There are many paths—paths of prayer, of study, of redirecting bodily energies in hatha yoga, of devotional singing in kirtan.

Many of us are strongly drawn to a path of service—the kind of service designed to alleviate the suffering of our fellow beings, service in deep harmony with the way of things, the dharma. When it is guided by the heart, such service feels like making love with God. Think of Mother Teresa seeing her beloved Jesus in all his distressing disguises.

Giving and receiving, depending on how they're done, can nourish people on both ends. Those who receive can help others feel graced and blessed to have the opportunity to serve. The art of receiving is a mindset that says, "I am a soul; you are a soul. We come together, and what roles we play is kind of irrelevant." Likewise, in serving, what you truly offer another being is your own being. That is how true healing occurs—your open heart allows the other person's heart to open. Then caregiving becomes a gift for everybody involved.

TAKING CARE OF DAD

Getting old, for example, can be a cause for more suffering, or it can be a state of grace. People who have been fiercely independent say, "I hate being dependent." On the other hand, I see people who are old and frail and need to be taken care of, but who are not at odds with themselves. They are so graceful and loving in their dependency that everybody who is taking care of them ends up feeling taken care of too.

I changed my father's diapers, as he had once changed mine. People said, "Oh, how disgusting." To him and me, it wasn't disgusting at all. It was a beautiful completion of a cycle. His mind had turned inward, and he was radiantly happy, peaceful, and relaxed. This was a guy who in his life had found happiness only in outer things, and now was radiating inner joy. Something in him transformed, and he turned into this other being. I was bathing him, and it was like washing the Buddha—incredible, blissed out, all the time. He didn't even recognize his former self. As he got older, my dad, who had been successful and active politically and socially, became very quiet. He just smiled a lot. I used to sit with him, hold his hand and watch the sunset. We had never done anything like that before. That is grace.

When you get to those edges where you say, "I can't handle that" or "I'm not going to do that," take a look at the mindset you are holding onto. There is the root of your suffering. That's where your mind is in relation to what is.

SEEING BEYOND SUFFERING

My friend Wavy Gravy is a living example of how to transform suffering. Among other roles, Wavy is a professional clown who visits children in the hospital. In full clown costume, complete with a big, round, red nose, he hangs out with children who are critically ill or dying. He blows bubbles. Sometimes he plays games with them. Sometimes he delights them with face paint. Sometimes they just hang out, and he shares and lightens their burdens.

Wavy says, "I don't know. Burnt skin or bald heads on little kids—what do you do? I guess you just face it. When the kids are really hurting so bad, so afraid and probably dying, and everybody's heart is breaking, face it. Face it and see what happens after that. See what to do next. I got the idea of traveling with popcorn. When a kid is crying, I dab the tears with the popcorn and pop it into my mouth or into his or hers. We sit around together and eat the tears."

When I was in India in 1971, there was tremendous devastation in Bangladesh. I wanted to help, and I went to Maharaj-ji to get his blessings. He said to me, "Can't you see it's all perfect?" I loved this man so deeply, but I remember feeling this was an obscenity. How could he say children starving to death was perfect? Yet this was a man of incredible compassion. He fed everybody, and he helped people all day all the time. He was saying I had lost my balance and had become so obsessed with the suffering that I couldn't see the greater picture.

This is about where you stand in your awareness, in a place that allows you to be with suffering in the world without closing your heart. If you close or armor your heart in order to be in the world, you become a crippled instrument for the healing of the universe. So you do all you can to relieve suffering and work to keep your heart open.

Another Indian saint, Swami "Papa" Ramdas, lived his life in continuous devotion to Rām. One night when he was sleeping outside by a river, he was being bitten by mosquitoes so much he couldn't sleep. His response was, "Oh Rām, thank you for bringing these mosquitoes and waking me so I could think about you all night."

Most of us are not quite ready for that. However, the recognition that suffering is a fire that purifies is an important concept. For a person who has not awakened, the game is to optimize pleasure and minimize suffering. As you become more aware, you recognize the reality of the Buddha's first Noble Truth: that existence on this plane involves suffering. The more conscious you become, the more you recognize that suffering is how the teaching you need in the moment is coming down. How you experience that suffering depends on your attachment, on how much you identify with what the Buddha describes as "the transient non-self," what we call the ego—who we think we are.

Consider what it's like to have a handicapped child—usually seen as a situation of sadness, suffering, and misfortune. But a different perception is that this soul has taken birth in this form with certain work to do. Part of that work is to recognize that he or she may not be fully understood or appreciated by the world around them. Your human heart as a parent wants to take away your child's suffering. But if you cultivate your spiritual awareness and meet this being as a soul, you can help him or her make contact with that part of their being that has nothing to do with a disability. As long as you see the child as being disabled, you are reinforcing that particular reality in which he or she is going to suffer. Meet the soul behind the disability. In that way, your work on yourself is an offering to your child.

I had a young friend, Kelly, whose body was quadriplegic. He had a misdiagnosed head injury when he was about nine years old. He was fully awake and brilliant, and at thirty-three years old, he was absolutely a delight. You could hold his hand over an alphabet board, and he could spell out words to communicate. Once when I was speaking before a group of doctors and holistic health healers, I had Kelly introduce me. About five hundred people were in the audience and Kelly was wheeled out onto the stage. They were all agape. Kelly spelled out, "RD says we are not our bodies. Amen."

HOW CAN WE HELP?

We often feel helpless in the face of suffering, especially the suffering of those close to us, and we wonder how we can help. Simple acts of kindness are so meaningful, like the quiet moments between people taking loving care of one another, or the support and kindness of friends and family expressing concern, offering help, prayers, and food. Food can be so much more than physical nourishment. Or perhaps you offer a flower from your garden, or just listen to the fears and feelings of someone who is suffering, so they know they are not alone. Sometimes just being there with an open heart and a presence grounded in peace and serenity is enough. These are reminders of grace that happen when you least expect them—reminders that nourish the soul.

COMPASSION

Bearing the unbearable is the deepest root of compassion in the world. When you bear what you think you cannot bear, who you think you are dies. You become compassion. You don't have compassion—you *are* compassion. True compassion goes beyond empathy to *being with* the experience of another. You become an instrument of compassion.

Your own suffering—be it loss, failure, grief, or physical pain—hurts like hell. Your heart may be broken. And yet, here you are.

You may have had an experience of suffering that burned deep into you and created a different quality of your being. You see the way that suffering forced your awakening. It's hard to imagine a spiritual curriculum in which Suffering 101 is not part of the course for becoming a full human being. It's a fierce teaching.

Part of that teaching is beginning to see through, or give up, seeking pleasure and avoiding pain, the pattern of desire and aversion that fastens you so intimately to *māya,* the illusion of separation. Something happens when you stop trying so hard to avoid suffering. When you wish it were different, you can't see how it is. There's a line in the Tao Te Ching that says, "Truth waits for eyes unclouded by longing." As you clear the mist of desire from your mirror, you start to reflect things as they are.

As you dwell more in loving awareness and see things as they truly are, you begin to expand beyond the boundaries of your separateness. You start to experience the outer world in a new way, so that instead of being in relationship to someone else, you become them. At that moment, the suffering of the universe is inside of you, not outside. True compassion arises out of the plane of consciousness where I am you, where you and I are one.

This is a Buddhist loving-kindness blessing, part of the Metta Meditation:

May all beings be free from danger.
May all beings be free from mental suffering.
May all beings be free from physical suffering.
May all beings know peace.
OM

Chapter 7

Content to Be

BEACH DAY

Once a week, I go to the beach on Maui for an ocean swim with a core crew of regulars. The rest of the group varies depending on who's visiting the island. We hang out on the beach for a while, and then we go in the water. Tom brings a bag of flowers and lovingly casts them on the water as we start to swim out toward the buoy marking the swimming area. I absolutely love being in the ocean. Sometimes we sing; often we laugh. We are just floating in Mother Ocean, surrounded by love. We play ball in the water. My ritual is to touch the float and say, "Oh buoy, oh buoy, oh buoy!" I have to be persuaded to return to the beach.

One day someone came up on the beach and asked what we were celebrating. One of the group said, "We're celebrating because it's today and we're together." We weren't being facetious. We meant to recognize the everyday sacredness of everything—*everything*.

Beach day is a perfect reflection of my feeling of contentment. You may be thinking it's easy to be content on a beach in Maui. It's true—it's a nice beach. But this is not about physical contentment. In yoga, *santosha,* or contentment, is a practice that helps you to quiet your mind and open your heart.

Contentment is one of the mindsets you use to direct your consciousness toward oneness. Oneness is the name of the game in yoga. True contentment is not just existential. It is an attitude of the soul rather than of the ego or personality. It is a view of life from the soul plane.

Love and compassion are emotions that arise from the soul. When you identify with your soul, you live in a loving universe. The soul loves everybody. It's like the sun. It brings out the beauty in each of us. You can feel that love radiating from your heart. When we are in that love, we enjoy just being wherever we are. There is a lot to be said for contentment like that.

Think of the kinds of experiences that give you a feeling of contentment. Maybe your contentment comes from being in nature, listening to the birds or the sound of the waves meeting the shore, looking at the sunset or the stars in the night sky, or contemplating a rose in the garden. Maybe it comes from singing or listening to music, sinking into a warm bath, or being touched in a way that eases the body. Maybe it comes from watching your child or being with your dog or cat. Maybe you experience it when looking into the eyes of a loved one. Those are experiences that touch your soul.

Contentment isn't high on the priority list in the West. We're all about achievement and consuming, getting more. Maybe we're afraid the wheels of progress and the economy will grind to a halt if everybody becomes content. I remember someone once accusing meditators of "bovine passivity." Living in the moment, being fully present, is anything but passive. But it does lead to a profound feeling that everything is just enough, a feeling of deep contentment.

Much of my sense of contentment comes from my relationship with Maharaj-ji and the constant remembrance of his presence in my life. Being in relationship with him is like having an infinitely deep pool of love and wisdom that always mirrors my deepest being.

And you are ever again the wave
sweeping through all things
RAINER MARIA RILKE, *BOOK OF HOURS*

I found in Maharaj-ji something that satisfied both my intellect and my heart. There was an intense degree of love, an oceanic feeling of love that pervaded the space he inhabited. There was an aura around him, a presence so powerful that you felt bathed and purified just by being anywhere near it. Even now, as I bring him into my heart, it does the same thing.

> *Since the day when I met with my Lord,*
> *There has been no end to the sport of our love.*
> *I see with eyes open and smile and behold His beauty everywhere.*
> *I utter his name and whatever I see it reminds me of Him.*
> *Whatever I do it becomes His worship.*
> . . .
> *Wherever I go I move round Him.*
> *All I achieve is His service.*
> *When I lie down, I lie prostrate at His feet.*
> . . .
> *Whether I rise or sit down I can never forget Him.*
> *For the rhythm of His music beats in my ears.*
> KABIR

My love for Maharaj-ji is my way of opening myself. He is constantly here, constantly reminding me of his presence. Moment by moment, I'm just hanging out with this being of consciousness, of love, of light, of presence.

These are some of the things Maharaj-ji said about love:

The worst punishment is to throw someone out of your heart.
You should not disturb anyone's heart.
Even if a person hurts you, give him love.
If you love God, you overcome all impurities.
You should love everyone as God. If you do not love each other, you cannot achieve your goal.
Christ said to love all beings as children of God and serve them.
Give everything to the poor, even your clothing. Give it all away.
Jesus gave everything away, even his body.

Someone asked Maharaj-ji how to meditate, and he replied, "Meditate the way Christ meditated." When asked how Christ did meditate, Maharaj-ji said, "He lost himself in love." He also said, "Christ was one with all beings and he had great love for all in the world. He was crucified so that his spirit could spread throughout the world. He was one with God. He sacrificed his body for the dharma. He never died. He never died. He is the Atmān living in the hearts of all. All beings are reflections of Christ.

"You will get pure love for Rām by the blessings of Christ. Hanuman and Christ are one. They are the same."

Maharaj-ji was asked what was the best method of meditation. He said, "Do as Jesus did and see God in everyone. Take pity on all and love all as God. When Jesus was crucified, he felt only love."

GETTING HIP

One day in 2009, I went to get a book, and I had an accident. I fell on my hip. There it was—a broken hip. I'm over eighty years old now, so I guess it comes with the territory. But that broken hip was my own fault. I'm in a wheelchair much of the time, and that day when I was transferring to the wheelchair, I didn't focus carefully, and I fell. The dilemma for me is that if I pay attention to my body full time, even when I am transferring, my consciousness doesn't get to be with my soul because I'm attending to my body, as most people do. I guess that inattention is a symptom of my separateness—if I were really living in the One, there'd be no difference between soul consciousness and body consciousness.

So I'm in the hospital getting my hip repaired. Hospitals are body oriented. They're body shops. To most of the hospital staff, I am the old guy in Room 322 with a broken hip. That's who I am in their professional view. Nurses and doctors are souls whose roles include seeing the problems of the body and treating them. So they must know, right?

The overwhelming mindset in a hospital is that we are our bodies. But aren't we also souls? Now, my view is that I am in this incarnation to learn about my true Self, to learn about my soul. Along the way I have also learned about strokes and broken hips. As I learned, you can think about them in many different ways.

From my point of view, the workings of the body are grist for the mill to get to the soul. It's tough work because these bodies really capture our attention. Learning to swim is nothing compared to learning to live from the soul plane.

In our minds the body is out there and the soul, the "I," is in here. To get to my soul, I have to turn my attention inward instead of outward. But I have to turn it selectively inward, because at the same time the body is demanding attention, and I better decide where my foot should go, or I am going to get myself killed. So I attend to my body when it's time to, and the rest of the time I work on being a soul.

The body and soul are like a coach and horses and a coachman. The horses are desires. The coachman is the ego, the "I" that controls the desires and looks where he's going (and makes sure the foot doesn't go in the wrong place). But inside the coach is a passenger. Who is riding in the coach? It's our soul. "Coachman, would you stop, please?" "Coachman, you are going a little too fast."

I am riding in my coach, and now and then my coach needs a grease job or a new bearing or a joint replaced. I'm in the coach shop for a hip joint, and they're the coach repair experts. That's fine as long as I know who I am—that I'm not the coach, that I am a passenger inside the coach riding along, merrily, merrily, merrily.

On the outside I am recovering from a hip replacement operation, but inside I am dancing. I look like an old fart, but I am dancing inside. And what a joyful, joyful dance! In India it's called the *lila,* the dance or the love play of the soul. And you can join in the *lila* anytime, because it's always going on. Here in this moment, it never stops.

Did I lose my soul in the hospital? Well, maybe I lost the connection with my soul for a while, but I didn't lose my soul. Where could it go? I'm still here. I have a new hip. I'm even hipper than I was.

ROLES TO SOULS

As we've discussed, within our consciousness are these different points of view. There's the ego and there's the soul, our spiritual self. They are two different planes of consciousness. From the spiritual vantage point, we are all souls who have come into these incarnations. We take birth, and this is our incarnation. Here we are, each of us an individual being.

When I used to travel back and forth from America to India, I would land in New Delhi and take a bus up to a village in the mountains. The people in that village knew they were souls. One was sweeping the road, and another was the governor. The governor was not just a governor, and the sweeper was not just busy being a sweeper. They had these roles for this incarnation, but they also identified themselves as souls. I'd go back to America, and when they opened the plane door in New York, everyone thought they were their roles. I'd go back and forth, roles to souls, souls to roles.

Because of the pull of the incarnation, we get so deeply into our roles that we forget we are souls. With all the sensations, emotions, and complications of being in a body, all the desires, we forget. We think, "I am a man. I am a woman. I am from California. I am a mother, a father, a widow, a child"—a something. "I've got to be something, don't I?"

Think of all the ways you identify yourself with what you do: "I am a teacher. I am a doctor, I'm a scientist. I'm a cook, a Jew or Christian or Muslim, a stockbroker. I'm an achiever. I am a spiritual seeker."—That one can carry you for years—"I am retired."

All that is the ego, who you think you are, the cluster of thoughts about how you identify yourself, thoughts about different roles that you play in society. When we meet someone we ask, "How do you do? And what do you do?" But is what you do the same as who you are?

Every one of our roles is a thought form. We confuse our souls with our roles. You don't see me as a soul. You see me as Ram Dass, as a body, a role. What does it matter whether I am a cellist, or a pilot, or a teacher? When you strip away the roles, this outer form is just the body. Who I am is just here. Instead of "How do you do?" how about, "How do you be?" Our inner being is beyond form.

When you live from your soul and your heart is open, you can awaken other souls. You go into a grocery store, and it's like a temple. Everybody is a soul. Some think they are customers; some think they work there. You get to the checkout, and your eyes lock for an instant with the clerk's. "Are you here? I'm here. Wow, a fellow soul!"

If you have children, your children are souls. They're just playing the roles of children, and you're in the mother or father role.

If you're with a dying person and you see them as a soul, that transition from ego to soul is easier to make. If, as a caregiver, you're identified with your soul, it is easy to see the dying person as a soul and to ease their transition.

JUST A MOMENT, PLEASE!

When we plumb the moment—this moment, not back then, not the future, but this moment—we get deeper and deeper and deeper into the universal heart of being. Finally, being in the moment blossoms into everything and nothing. It's all in this moment. This moment is always here. Now is eternal.

That joy you get from being completely in the moment brings contentment. Contentment, as a practice, is different from satisfaction. It's not a feeling of accomplishment from doing something. Contentment is just being complete in the moment.

Burrow into the moment. Then you're in the moment, and here we are in the moment. If something is taking me out of the moment, I'll say, "What am I doing here?" or "What is it that blocks my contentment? It's raining. Doesn't rain make me content? The flowers are so grateful, and the rain is just beautiful, little drops on the window. They're each like little globes. And now I'm content."

I'm content to take a nap without thinking I should be doing something else. I'm even content to have a broken hip that's healing. It's part of the body growing old. But *I* am just here.

When I first traveled to India in 1966, I was just another Westerner visiting a foreign country. I was with a friend traveling in a Land Rover. We had canned tuna fish and Vivaldi tapes, beds, and all kinds of Western amenities. We looked out through the windows at this foreign culture.

When we came to Benares, the holy city where Hindus go to die, people were walking the streets with leprosy and all kinds of illnesses, just waiting to die. They each had a pouch, a little bundle of cloth, that held the coins for their funeral pyre, to pay for the wood to burn their body.

As we drove through this city, I thought, "These people have no hospital. They have no support system. They're just waiting to die." These depressing thoughts and the ubiquitous poverty made me feel awful. When we got to the hotel, I hid under the bed.

I visited Benares again six months later. It was the same scene, but in those six months I had been living in a Hindu temple up in the Himalayas under my guru's tutelage. Now, instead of being just a Westerner, I was maybe a Hind-Jew or a little Buddh-ish. I began to see that Benares was a city of incredible joy, even though it held incredible physical suffering. Instead of seeing "those poor people," instead of being overwhelmed and pushing away their pain, I could stop to look in their eyes.

I saw two things. First, they looked at me with compassion, as if I were a hungry ghost, a homeless spirit wandering from place to place. And second, they themselves were content.

How could they be content amidst all that suffering? They were content because if you are a Hindu and you die in Benares by the holy river Ganges, Shiva whispers in your ear and liberates you. These beings were in the right place at the right time. They were dying in the perfect place for a Hindu to die.

Their contentment really got to me. How could they be so content? It conflicted with all my Western values. My Western life had always been about achievement, wanting, desiring, doing more, getting more. I always felt as if I were in the wrong place at the wrong time because there must be something better. I was forever collecting the next achievement. But those people in Benares had something I hadn't been able to collect: contentment.

ALL YOU NEED IS . . .

If I am in my soul, when I look at others, I see their souls. I still see the individual differences—men and women, rich and poor, attractive and unattractive, and all that stuff. But when we recognize each other as souls, we are seeing each other as aspects of the One. Love is the emotion of merging, of becoming One. Love is a way of pushing through into the One.

We treat love and hate and the other emotions like they are all on the same level, but they're not. Hate, fear, lust, greed, jealousy—all that comes from the ego. Only love comes from the soul. When you identify with your soul, you live in a loving universe. The soul loves everybody. It's like the sun. It brings out the beauty in each of us. You can feel it in your heart.

In those early days of being with Maharaj-ji, he would tell me repeatedly, "Ram Dass, love everyone and tell the truth." At that time I could only touch that place for occasional moments. I was living most of the time on the ego plane. I could love almost everyone for short periods of time, but the truth was that I did not love everyone. There was that day when I was so angry with everyone and Maharaj-ji came up to me, nose to nose, looked me in the eye, and said, "Ram Dass, love everyone *and* tell the truth." He was telling me to take a different path and *become* a soul. What he was saying is that when I can relate from that soul plane of consciousness, which is who I really *am*, I will love everyone. That *is* my truth. It's only taken me forty years to figure it out.

Learn the art of taking your stand on the Truth within. When you live in this Truth, the result is the fusion of the mind and the heart and the end of all fears and sorrow. It is not a dry attainment of mere power or intellectual knowledge. A love which is illumined by the intuitive wisdom of the spirit will bless your life with ever-renewing fulfillment and never-ending sweetness.
MEHER BABA, *LIFE AT ITS BEST*

You can stay in touch with your soul by dwelling in the moment. Soul is centered in your heart. It is the heart-mind. Do your daily acts with love. That's what the soul can do. When you are identified with your soul, you not only reflect God's light, but you also become a mirror for others to find their souls. The only goal a soul has is to satisfy God and become one with the Beloved.

Everything is as it should be. I say that because I've surrendered, surrendered to the One. The One makes this moment perfectly fulfilled—and I am quiet and peaceful inside. Go inside for peace, go inside for compassion, go inside for wisdom, go inside for joy, go inside for love.

MEDITATION: I AM LOVING AWARENESS

The Atmān, the universal soul within all, manifests within you as your individual soul, that part of you that is wisdom, compassion, joy, love, and peace. Start by quieting down and going inside to your spiritual heart space. Allow yourself to sink deeper and deeper into your soul. Concentrate on the middle of your chest and allow this phrase to reverberate in this heart space: "I am loving awareness. I am loving awareness. . . ." Allow it to become part of you. Then with grace you will become just loving awareness.

Use your breath to continue centering: in, out, in, out. The movement of air at the nostrils at the tip of your nose or the rise and fall of your diaphragm in your belly are good places to keep centering on your breathing. As your thoughts subside into the ocean of the breath, keep bringing your concentration to the middle of your heart space. That point is your spiritual heart. And that loving awareness *is* you—it's the real you, because you *are* awareness. Now, you can be aware of your eyes and what they see; you can be aware of the ears and what they hear; you can be aware of your skin and what it feels. You can be aware of your mind and the river of thoughts that flows from your mind. Thoughts, thoughts, thoughts . . .

Some of those thoughts are positive; some are negative; some are about you and about others. Some of them are judging thoughts. But you stay identified with loving awareness in your heart, in the heart center. "I am loving awareness. I am loving awareness. I am loving awareness. I am loving awareness."

Awareness is not a thing. We can label it, but it is not the words. You *are* loving awareness. So is Christ. So is Krishna. So is Buddha. So is Maharaj-ji. They are loving awareness, and so are you. Loving awareness is one—one loving awareness.

Each of us is a finger of the hand of universal awareness. Loving awareness is in everybody; everybody is in loving awareness. Wars and disagreements, separate nations, those are the games we play. Yet we are loving awareness. We are individuals, but we're not. We are all God. You are an individual, and you are also part of the whole. You are loving awareness, and when you finally get to *be* loving awareness, just *be* loving awareness.

BEING LOVE NOW

I honor the light in all of us. The more I love God, the more I love the forms of God, which are all forms. Living from the soul is very much a heart-center journey. I get on a bus, and by the time I get off, I feel like I have met intimate family members I've known all my life. We're all in love with one another. To live in your spiritual heart with the degree of openness it entails, trust in the One. In that loving awareness, you are not as vulnerable as you would be in the ego, where you think you are separate from others.

> *How did the rose ever open its heart*
> *And give to this world all of its beauty?*
> *It felt the encouragement of light against its being,*
> *Otherwise we all remain too frightened.*
> HAFIZ, "HOW DID THE ROSE?" TRANSLATED BY DANIEL LADINSKY

How does one become loving awareness? If I change my identification from the ego to the soul, then as I look at people, they all appear like souls to me. I change from my head, the thought of who I am, to my spiritual heart, which is a different sort of awareness—feeling directly, intuiting, loving awareness. It's changing from a worldly outer identification to a spiritual inner identification. Concentrate on your spiritual heart, right in the middle of your chest. Keep repeating the phrase, "I am loving awareness. I am loving awareness. I am loving awareness."

The object of our love is love itself. It is the inner light in everyone and everything. Love is a state of being.

You begin to love people because they just *are.* You see the mystery of the Divine in form. When you live in love, you see love everywhere you look. You are literally *in* love with everyone you look at.

When that starts to happen, as you fall in love with everyone you meet, you may think you want to collect them all. So you get one and you say, "Let's nest." And you get furniture and drapes and you make a nest. You go out to the supermarket to get tofu and beer, and you look into the eyes of the person at the checkout counter. The eyes are the windows of the soul, so you look, and there's your Beloved too. Now what are you going to do? You've already got one at home. Do you say, "Have you considered a ménage à trois?"

You have to graduate from a deprivation to an abundance model. It's abundant because you *are* it; you are radiating love wherever you go. As you become love, when you walk down the street, everyone is the most beautiful person all over again. You look and appreciate. You may meet another's eyes, and you both recognize the love, but you don't have to do anything about it.

The art form of relationship is to realize that every relationship you are in—every relationship at every moment—is a vehicle for awakening love. And it's up to you. The Beloved is everywhere.

There was a moment when I was on a lecture tour and I was staying at a funky motel. It was one of those really plastic places. I arrived and I went into my room and I sat down and I was starting to set up my little puja table on the plastic bureau. I was moving the hotel menu and stuff and sitting there, and it was kind of depressing. I thought, "Well, a few more weeks and this tour will be over, and I can go home." Then I saw the pain that thought was creating.

I got up, and I walked out of the room, closed the door, walked down the hall, turned around, came back, unlocked the door and yelled, "I'm home!" I came in and I sat down and I looked and I thought to myself, "You know, I wouldn't particularly have decorated this way, but what the hell."

If I am not at home anywhere in the universe, I've got a problem. If I say I can only be home here, but not there, what is home? Home is where the heart is. Home is the quality of presence. It's the quality of being. Home is always here.

Quiet your mind; let go of molds and models and thought forms. Open your heart and let your thoughts and emotions get consumed by the moment until you become just pure presence. Now you are living in the Tao, and it is with you wherever you go.

> *Don't go outside your house to see flowers.*
> *My friend, don't bother with that excursion.*
> *Inside your body there are flowers.*

One flower has a thousand petals.
That will do for a place to sit.
Sitting there you will have a glimpse of beauty
inside the body and out of it,
before gardens and after gardens.
KABIR, "A PLACE TO SIT"

When you and I rest together in loving awareness, we swim together in the ocean of love. Remember, it's always right here. Enter into the flow of love with a quiet mind and see all things with love as part of yourself.

THE WHEEL OF ILLUSION

A soul takes a human birth in order to have a series of experiences through which it will awaken out of its illusion of separateness. This physical experience of being incarnated is the curriculum, and the purpose of the course is to awaken us from the illusion that we are the incarnation. Spiritual practices are tools to help us accomplish these goals.

You start from innocence and you return to innocence. A sage was asked, "How long have we been on this journey?" He replied, "Imagine a mountain three miles wide, three miles high, and three miles long. Once every hundred years, a bird flies over the mountain, holding a silk scarf in its beak, which it brushes across the surface of the mountain. In the time it takes for the scarf to wear away the mountain, that's how long we've been doing this."

We are on an inevitable course of awakening. If you understand that message deeply, it allows you to enter into your spiritual practices from a different perspective, one of patience and timelessness. You do your practices not out of a sense of duty or because you *think* you should, but because you know in your soul there really is nothing else you would rather do.

In Sanskrit this is called *vairagya,* a state of weariness with worldly desire where only the desire for spiritual fulfillment is left. The spiritual pull is the last desire, one that really grabs you, but that dissolves on its own because you dissolve in the process. The Tao says, "In the end you will be like the valley which is the favorite resort of the Way." You become receptive, become soft, become open, become attuned, become quiet. You become the ocean of love.

> *The soul is made of love, and must ever strive to return to love. It can never find rest nor happiness in other things. It must lose itself in love.*
> MECHTHILD OF MAGDEBURG

> *In the end, all our other desires merge in the immense longing to have no barrier between us and our real Beloved.*
> EKNATH EASWARAN

Time is a box formed by thoughts of the past and future. When there is only the immediate *now*—when you're not dwelling in the past or anticipating the future, but you are just right here, right now—you're outside of time. Dwelling in the moment is dwelling in the soul, which is eternal presence.

When we're outside of time, there's no subject or object; it's all just here. The thinking mind deals only with subject and object. But from within *here now,* you watch time go by. You are not being in time. You *be,* and time goes by, as if you were standing on a bridge and watching it all go by.

Ours is a journey toward simplicity, toward quietness, toward a kind of joy that is not in time. In this journey out of time to "NowHere," we are leaving behind every model we have had of who we thought we were. This journey involves a transformation of our being so that our thinking mind becomes our servant rather than our master. It's a journey that takes us from primary identification with our psyche to identification with our souls, then to identification with God, and ultimately beyond any identification at all.

Life is an incredible curriculum in which we live richly and passionately as a way of awakening to the deepest truths of our being. As a soul, I have only one motive: to merge with God. As a soul, I live in the moment, in each rich and precious moment, and I am filled with contentment.

> *May the Blessings of God*
> *Rest upon you.*
> *May His Peace*

Abide with you
May His Presence
Illuminate your heart
Now and forever more.
SUFI PRAYER

Chapter 8

Practicing Practicing

ARE THERE BENEFITS in creating a daily spiritual practice? On the level where we are pure souls, where we are simply loving awareness, it doesn't matter. There is just being here now. Living fully in the moment, there is no practice, only being. If you have become stable in this presence, ignore this chapter. You are already here.

On the other hand, if your mind still wanders, you may find some benefit in using these practices to bring you back to your Self, to be more present, to open your heart, to learn to live from your spiritual heart. Practices are designed to put you back in touch with your true nature, the Self, to polish the mirror of your mind and heart so they truly reflect the spirit.

Most of us are enmeshed in the world, and we get lost very easily in the stuff of life. A daily practice is very useful to keep reminding you, to keep pulling you back and waking you up again, giving you a chance to see how you got lost the day before and to keep putting what's happening to you in the world back into a spiritual perspective.

For instance, I read a little passage in the morning when I wake up. I have books next to my bed, and I'll just pick one up and start the day reading a *sloka,* a passage from a holy book, or a little quote from a saint, and it will just start me remembering, reminding me what the game is about.

You can tune to the spirit through a variety of practices. Look to each method to keep opening you in its own unique way. At the beginning, when you're trying different methods, be generous with yourself. There will be a method that will fit your unique karma. If you come to a practice with a pure heart and a yearning to be free, it will reflect back the purity of your aspiration.

Spiritual practice isn't a way to achieve something or to get somewhere else. You're already here. You do spiritual practices because you do spiritual practices, not to get to some other state, but to get in touch with who you already are, to clear the dust from the mirror, to come more fully into the present moment. Whether you will be free and enlightened now or in ten thousand births is not the point. What else is there to do? You can't stop doing them anyway. Once you awaken to the possibility of the universe within, it's like a gravitational force.

Don't get trapped in your expectations. Spiritual practices can themselves become obstacles if you become too attached to them. Use these methods as consciously as you can, knowing that if they are truly working, eventually they will self-destruct.

MAKING A SACRED SPACE

Create a quiet corner in your home for practice—an Om home, a launching pad to the infinite, a meditation seat, a shrine to your inmost Self.

In India, worship is called *puja,* and a puja table or puja room is a sacred space for meditation, worship, prayer, reading holy books, reflection, centering, doing mantra or chanting. It is a place for remembering your Self, getting in touch with your guru, or just a source of spiritual comfort. It can be a space for doing devotional rituals or for making offerings of love, a flower, incense, food, or just gratitude.

Make this space simple and pure: perhaps with a mat, a candle, some incense, a picture of a realized being you feel connected to—Buddha or Christ, Rām or Krishna, or your guru. Create a seat where you can sit comfortably, with your back straight. Zen Buddhists use a zafu and *zabuton*, a meditation cushion and pad. Use whatever helps you sit comfortably—a bench or a chair if you need it. This is *your* sacred space.

Make your puja table a beautiful offering that reflects what is spiritually meaningful for you. It can be in a corner of a room, in a closet, or if you have the space, in a separate room. You may wish to cover the table with a cloth. A fresh flower as an offering to your Beloved adds to the sweetness. Holy statues, photos of loved ones you wish to bless, prayers written for family or friends who are suffering or sick, may help open your heart. If you are having problems with someone, try putting their picture on your puja table so that after meditating you can bring them into the Light. Keep holy books nearby, handy for daily use.

If you already have an established puja table, know that you can never have too many sacred spaces. You can always deepen your spiritual practices. Let Spirit permeate your life. Surround yourself with images of the Divine, reminders of what is really important in life. Let them help quiet your mind, open your heart, and bring inner peace.

You can create small altars or shrines at your desk or in your computer space, on a countertop, at the entryway of your home, on the door of the refrigerator. Create a sanctuary in the garden, at your doorstep, on the patio or deck, on the dashboard of your car. Spiritualize your life from the outside, but know the real work is within.

MORNING PRACTICE

As water wears away stone, so daily sadhana, or spiritual practice, will thin the veil of illusion.

For starters, consider getting up a half hour earlier to allow time for your spiritual practices.

Remove your shoes when you approach your puja table. Invest this space with a spirit of love, reverence, devotion, and gratitude. Light some incense. Connect with the images on your puja and settle into just *being here now*! Let go of everything other than being present in this sacred space.

If, as I mentioned, you can start your day in a conscious manner by reading a passage from a holy book, you can bring it to mind as an occasional reminder throughout the day. You might want to play some peaceful music or chanting, or do some singing or chanting yourself.

THE DAILY NOW

Keeping a journal helps you to have a reflection of your thoughts and will give you a place to process and record teachings, feelings, or insights that occur on this journey. At times I've kept a diary of how often during the day that I have lost it and got caught in the drama of it all and started to take the illusion of *māya* as real. I'd just make a list and then look at the patterns of those lists over days. They showed me the nature of my desire systems. They showed me what it was that I made real.

You might want to record your reflections on the Words from Realized Beings section at the end of this chapter and how they apply to your life. As you go through the day, notice how often you are truly present in the moment, when your heart is open, when it closes down.

When you act in harmony with dharma, a quality of equanimity comes into everything you do. Witness your life, your actions; observe your motivations for doing things, your desires. See what leads to anger, fear, greed, lust, love. Pull back. Do your meditative practices. Watch the world go by from inside your spiritual heart.

Lose it. Examine it. Quiet down again. Lose it again. Write in your journal. Watch what makes you lose it every time. Just watch it all. No judging. Really get to know yourself.

Note what happens to your spiritual center in your relationships. Your needs and desires may be giving someone else power over you. Someone else's ability to take you out of your equanimity has to do with your attachment and the clinging of mind. That's your work on yourself.

MEDITATION

Meditation is basic spiritual practice for quieting the mind and getting in touch with our deeper Self, the spirit. Meditation provides a deeper appreciation of the interrelatedness of all things and the part each person plays. The simple rules of this game are honesty with yourself about where you are in your life and learning and listening to hear how it is. Meditation is a way of listening more deeply, so you hear how it all is from a more profound place. Meditation enhances your insight, reveals your true nature, and brings you inner peace.

A meditation practice is extremely useful in clearing stuff away and letting you see how your mind keeps creating your universe. The ego will keep you occupied with its endless story line of thought forms. Just keep watching them until they dissolve.

Most traditions require a regular practice in order to progress, to get ahead. On the other hand, there are traditions in which no regular practice is required and people do fine, so I can't say it is necessary. But I certainly find it useful, and I encourage other people to do it.

Regularly practicing meditation, even when you don't feel like it, will help you see how your thoughts impose limits and color your existence. Resistances to meditation are your mental prisons in miniature.

It's delicate, because you have to practice from the place of really remembering why you're doing it, with some joy and appreciation. If you go into it with, "Oh, I gotta do my practice," the practice will eventually clean that resistance out of you, but I don't necessarily feel that's a good thing. That's what happens to people when they have to go to church every Sunday. I would rather push you away from spiritual practices until you're so hungry for them that you really want to do a practice, rather than give you a sense that you ought to do the practice or that you're a bad person if you don't do it, because you will end up hating the whole business. In the long run I don't think it will be good for you. Spiritual practice is wonderful if you want to do it. And if you don't, don't.

There are many different forms of meditation from a host of spiritual traditions. I will share with you some of the methods that have been most effective for me over the years. They include *Vipāssana* (or insight) meditation from the Southern Buddhist tradition, mantra from Hindu bhakti devotional practice (including how to practice mantra with a mala, or rosary), and guru kripa (grace of the guru) meditation.

Remember the story of a Westerner arriving at the ashram in India and asking Maharaj-ji how to meditate? Maharaj-ji became quiet and closed his eyes. After a few moments, a tear trickled down his cheek, and he said, "Meditate the way Christ meditated. He lost himself in Love. Christ lives in the hearts of all beings. He never died. He never died. "

Lose yourself in love.

When you are with someone you love very much,
you can talk and it is pleasant, but the reality
is not in the conversation.
It is simply in being together.
Meditation is the highest form of prayer.
In it you are so close to God that you don't need to say a thing
It's just great to be together.
SWAMI CHETANANDA

Vipāssana Meditation

Vipāssana, or insight meditation, is a fundamental Buddhist meditation, drawn from Southern Buddhism. The focus or primary object of this meditation is the breath, and the beginning practice is just following the breath. Concentration on the breath is called *anapanna,* and it is just bringing you right here, now, through the breath. Everyone breathes. We all have our individual differences but we are all breathing in and breathing out.

Sit comfortably, with your body as straight as is comfortable, your head, neck, and chest aligned. Take two or three intentional slow, deep breaths, and close your eyes.

Focus on your breath going in and your breath coming out. Two ways you can do this are:

- By focusing on the muscle in the solar plexus, which every time you breathe in, moves in one direction, and every time you breathe out, moves in another direction—rising, falling, rising, falling.
- By focusing on the inside of your nostrils at the tip of your nose—as the air goes by, you will feel a slight whisper of air on the in breath, and as the air goes out, you will feel a slight whisper of air on the out breath.

Use whichever of those two spots is easiest for you to do. Pick one focus, either the rising and falling of the muscle in your abdomen or the air going by the tip of your nose, and stay with it for a period of at least fifteen minutes.

You are like a gatekeeper at the gate. Cars go in and cars go out. You don't need to see where they go. You just notice the breath going in, breathing in, and the breath going out, breathing out. Your job is solely to focus your awareness on your primary object of the breath in the gentlest way possible.

Your awareness is going to wander; it is going to be grabbed by many stray thoughts. You'll sit down and you'll say, "Breathing in, breathing out" or "Rising, falling." Then the thought will come, "This will never work." Now you can either take that thought "This will never work" and immediately go off on another train of thought, and even though you have instructions to follow, you just ignore them and then the meditation time is over. That's okay. Or at some point when you get tired of that, you can say, "Gee, all I was going to do for these fifteen minutes was watch my breath. This is just another thought. Maybe I'll just let it go, and I'll go back to watching my breath." See, that's a strategy for gently bringing your mind back to the breath, for coming back to your awareness.

The art is to not get violent with your other thoughts. Don't try to push them away. Don't feel guilty because you are thinking them. They're just thoughts. Very gently, again and again, simply bring your awareness back to the primary object of meditation: breathing in, breathing out. Just keep coming back to the focus of your meditation, back to the breath, back to awareness of the breath.

Whether your breathing gets fast or slow doesn't matter; just notice it. Don't try to change it, but just notice it. You are merely remaining aware: the gatekeeper watching the gate open and close. Any sounds, smells, or sensations, just let them come and let them go and bring your awareness back to either rising and falling or breathing in and breathing out.

If your mind wanders, just notice it, then very gently bring it back to breathing in and breathing out or rising and falling. Wherever your mind is now, just notice where it is and very gently bring it back to rising and falling or breathing in and breathing out. If it helps to think to yourself "Breathing in, breathing out" with each breath, that is perfectly okay. If it helps to count breaths, try counting to ten, counting each in- and out-breath cycle as one, and then start over. If your mind wanders off in the middle, start over. Sometimes it can be really hard to get to ten! But don't judge yourself, don't get frustrated, there's no success or failure—only your awareness of the breath.

All the sounds, everything that comes into your ears, just notice them as more thoughts and come back to your breath. There is nothing you need to think about now other than breathing in and breathing out or rising and falling.

Notice the shape and form as the breath goes by—the beginning, middle, and end of the in breath; the space in between; the beginning, middle, and end of the out breath; and again the space.

If you experience agitation or confusion or boredom or bliss or anything, just see it as another thought. Notice it and bring your awareness back to rising and falling or breathing in and breathing out.

If you begin to doze, take a few deep intentional breaths. Rising and falling or breathing in and breathing out. All the feelings in your body—the sounds, the sensations, the tastes, the smells, the sights—just notice them coming and going and bring your awareness back to the primary object of meditation.

Firm your seat, head straight, rising and falling or breathing in and breathing out. If you are getting to the end of your sit, use these last minutes consciously. There is no beginning and no end. Every breath is the first and last.

Gently but firmly each time your mind wanders, bring it back to rising and falling or breathing in and breathing out. Be vigilant but gentle. Bring the awareness back to the basic primary object of meditation, the breath.

If your mind becomes agitated in the course of the day, bring it back to the breath, rising and falling, breathing in and breathing out.

OM

Meditation on the Guru

Imagine a realized being standing before you, someone to whom you feel particularly attuned, such as Christ, Mary, Mohammed, Rām, Hanuman, Anandamayi Ma, or your guru. This being is radiant, luminous, with eyes that are filled with compassion. You feel this being radiating the wisdom that comes from an intimate harmony with the universe.

It is just so incredibly gentle and beautiful to start a dialogue of love with a being who *is* love. Sit in your meditation area and gaze at a picture of a being whose love is pure, whose love reflects the light of God. Experience that love flowing back and forth between you and the picture. Just open yourself and surrender.

See yourself reflected in those compassionate, nonjudging eyes, and allow yourself to open more and more. This is your Beloved. Sit before this being, or imagine such a being sitting in your heart. Just be with that being and return the love. Despite all of the impurities to which you cling, despite all your feelings of unworthiness, such a being loves you unconditionally. It's OK to carry on imaginary conversations with this being; the exchange opens you to compassion, tranquility, warmth, patience—to all the qualities of a free being.

This interpersonal quality of devotional meditation allows you to start from your psychological need to love and to be loved and to bring it into the presence of wisdom, compassion, and peace. When you are with a being who embodies these qualities, they rub off, and you feel more evolved, even to the point of recognizing the radiant light within yourself. Acknowledging your own beauty allows you to open even more to the Beloved, until finally the lover and Beloved merge, and you find that what you had seen outwardly as perfection in your Beloved is a mirror of your own inner beauty.

Ultimately you become that kind of love. You're living in that space and don't need anybody to turn you on to love because you *are* it, and everybody who comes near you drinks of it. And as you become more and more the statement of love, you fall into love with everyone.

Mantra

A mantra is a repeated prayer, words, a holy name, or a sacred sound or sounds. It's like a tape loop going on inside that reminds me of who I *am*. It's like a niche in the wall where the candle flame never flickers. It always brings me right back into to my heart, into the eternal present.

A mantra can be a name or names of God, in Sanskrit or English or Spanish or whatever language you know. It is usually recited silently in the mind, though at times you may want to say it aloud or subvocally, still keeping it internalized and without intruding on other people's psychic space. Sanskrit is interesting because it is based on seed syllables, or *bij* mantras, that set up vibrational fields through sound. They work even when recited silently, reverberating within.

Some mantras are more conceptual. All mantra works by repetition. Practiced consistently, mantra has the ability to steady the mind and transform consciousness. Mantra should be repeated frequently. It can be repeated any time, any place—when you're walking, taking a shower, washing the dishes, waiting in line for the movies.

In Buddhism, the word "mantra" means "mind protecting." A mantra protects the mind by preventing it from going into its usual mechanical habits, which often are not our optimal conscious perspective. Mantra is a powerful spiritual practice for centering and for letting go of strong emotions, such as fear, anxiety, and anger. The more you practice mantra, the more it becomes a part of you. When you need it on the psychological level—for example, when you feel afraid—using your witness, you notice the fear and replace the fear with your mantra. This will occur naturally once mantra becomes an established practice. Mantra is a daily reminder of the presence of the Divine within ourselves and in the universe.

Mahatma Gandhi said, "The mantra becomes one's staff of life and carries one through every ordeal. It is no empty repetition. For each repetition has a new meaning, carrying you nearer and nearer to God."

Keep repeating your mantra consciously until it becomes a strong habit. Go for a walk and say the mantra all the time you are walking. Notice everything but keep the mantra going. Keep realizing that being with God is your focus—and therefore everything you see is part of God.

Maharaj-ji said, "The best form in which to worship God is in all forms." Everyone you meet is Rām, who has come to teach you something. Mantra is remembering that place in the heart. Rām, Rām, Rām. Say it, mouth it, think it, feel it in your heart. You are continually meeting the Beloved and merging into perfection.

The Divine is present in the soul of all living beings and throughout the universe. God has been called by different names in different ages, countries, and religions. According to the Hindu view, an avatar is an incarnation of divine consciousness in human form. An avatar takes birth at a time when spiritual teaching is needed to establish new pathways for realization. Rām, Krishna, Buddha, and Jesus are all avatars in the Hindu view. Their names evoke divine power and are often used in mantra.

Once you choose a mantra and establish a practice, it is a good idea not to change mantras too much. If you stick with the same mantra, the practice will become deeper. Following are some mantras; you can select one that feels right for you or find one from a tradition that feels comfortable to you. Use whatever name you associate with the Divine.

My guru, Neem Karoli Baba, used *Rām,* and he often could be seen mouthing, "Rām, Rām, Rām, Rām, Rām . . ." Rām (or Rāma) in the *Rāmayana* is a being of great light, love, compassion, wisdom, and power, who lives in perfect harmony with the dharma, the One. Rām is the essence of who you are when you realize your true Self, the Atmān.

Sri Rām, Jai Rām, Jai, Jai, Rām ("Beloved Rām, I honor you")

If you use *Rām* when you meditate, say/think/feel *Rām* on the out breath. The out breath is the breath you will experience at the end of your life. Associate it with love, mercy, compassion, bliss, letting go. Train yourself into this Rām mind.

Another option is the *maha-mantra* ("great mantra") to both Krishna and Rām:

Hare Krishna, Hare Krishna,
Krishna, Krishna, Hare, Hare.
Hare Rāma, Hare Rāma,
Rāma, Rāma, Hare, Hare

Krishna represents many aspects of human love: parental love, romantic love, and love between friends. His instructions to Arjuna in the Bhagavad Gita are a complete teaching on living life as a spiritual practice.

Om is a sacred sound mantra, one of the bij (seed) syllables mentioned earlier, sometimes called the sound of the universe. It's very primordial—think, "In the beginning was the word, and the word was God."

Om Namah Shivaya ("I bow to Shiva.")

Other mantras from Buddhism are:

Om mani padme hum ("I bow to the jewel in the lotus of the heart.")

Om Tare Tu Tare Ture Swaha ("to the Mother in the form of Tara.")

A mantra from the Greek Christian tradition, in the Philokalia:

Lord Jesus, Son of God, have mercy on me, a sinner.

Mantra can be practiced with a mala, a string of prayer beads. In the West, a mala is commonly called a rosary. A mala has 108 beads, plus a larger guru bead. A wrist mala has 27, 36, or 54 beads, plus a guru bead. All of these numbers—108, 54, 36, and 27—are sacred numbers in numerology, with digits that add up to nine. The mala is an external aid to doing mantra. You recite the mantra as you pass the beads through your fingers. The feeling of the beads moving through your fingers is a wonderful centering device.

In the traditional way I was taught to use a mala; you use your right hand, passing each bead between the thumb and the third finger, bead by bead, moving the beads toward you. With each bead repeat the name of Rām, or whatever your mantra is. Proceed to the guru bead, pause, and bring your guru or teacher to mind. Then turn the beads around and go the other way. Do not complete the circle. That helps you mark each cycle of 108.

Swami Ramdas, a devout Indian saint of the last century whose life revolved around listening to the will of Rām to guide his every activity, tells us, referring to mantra and kirtan (devotional chanting), "People do not know what the Name of God can do. Those who repeat it constantly alone know its power. It can purify our mind completely. . . . The Name can take us to the summit of spiritual experience."

SILENCE

Practicing silence will manifest in calmness and clarity of mind, more energy, and your enhanced ability to hear others with deeper understanding. Silence is part of the ongoing exercise of developing the witness. Notice how your mind interprets the world around you. If possible, set aside some time in your day or a weekend day to be in silence. Explain to family and friends your intention to be silent, so you will have their support in your efforts. But remember that it's just an exercise and don't make a big deal out of it. There is the external silence of not talking, and there is the deeper silence of a quiet mind.

BLESSING FOOD

Before I eat, I bless my food. For many people, saying grace in childhood was a time of impatience, when adults were controlling the situation, but I've discovered that it can become a moment to reawaken a living truth.

When I get food, I hold the food up or sit with my hands touching my plate, and I say a blessing. Sometimes in a restaurant I just quietly go inward; I don't have to make a big production out of it or stop other people from eating. I just think about God for a moment, and I realize that this whole ritual of praying over food is part of all form. It's part of law; it's part of the universe. The bowl of oatmeal I'm praying over is part of God, as is the farmer who grew it, the cook who prepared it, and I, who am making this prayer, offering it up. We're all part of God. The hunger the oatmeal will quiet, those pangs in my stomach, the fire of desire that will consume this food, these are also part of God. I begin to sense the oneness of everything; I start to experience a place of quiet understanding. The more deeply I appreciate the oneness that is the source of the food, the hunger, my belly, the more I become one with it all.

In India I learned a prayer to remind me of this oneness, a way to offer food and to bring me home:

Brahmarpanam Brahma Havir
Brahmagnau Brahmana Hutam
Brahmaiva Tena Ghantavyam
Brahmakarma Samadhina

The act of offering is God (Brahman).
The offering itself (the food) is God.
He/she who offers is God, and the sacred fire (which cooked the food
and receives the offering) is God.
He/she attains to God, who, in all actions, is absorbed in God.

Next time you are waiting for food to be served and are feeling impatient or hungry, use the time to think of God. Then when you receive the food, say a blessing and let it remind you that you and the food are one. Then eat. Rituals can become automatic or they can take you deeper. Over time this ritual, for me, has become a living connection to the Divine and my at-one-ment with everything manifest in the universe.

KIRTAN

In India, kirtan is chanting the names of God, a devotional practice that both opens your heart and quiets your mind. Much of what was said above about mantra applies to kirtan, which may use the same names or phrases, but you can also do kirtan together with others, with music.

In *Glimpses of Divine Vision,* the Indian saint Swami Ramdas says, "Devotion to God who is seated in the hearts of us all is the one path that leads the struggling soul to the haven of perfect peace and joy. . . . Devotion sweetens life. . . . Devotion means loving remembrance of God. Blessed indeed is the heart which adores the Lord and are the lips which utter His nectar-like name."

Krishna Das, one of Maharaj-ji's devotees, has been leading kirtan in the West for many years. He says, "Chanting is a way of getting in touch with yourself. It's an opening of the heart and letting go of the thoughts passing through the mind. It deepens the channel of grace, and it's a way of being present in the moment." Here is how he describes the practice:

> What we're singing is the repetition of the Divine Names, the Hindu names of God. Usually when you call someone's name you know who you're talking to. When we give something a name, like a baby's name or if you get a truck and it's a Chevy, we know that name defines the person or thing for us and the name aims our attention at it. With kirtan it's a little different.
>
> They say these Divine Names come from a place within us, a place that's before thought, before emotion, before anything to do with concepts or conceptual thinking. And these Names have been given to us or revealed to us by beings who, from their deeper experience, became aware of the names within themselves.
>
> Maharaj-ji used to say over and over again, *"Rām nām karnay se, sub pura ho jata,"* or that from repeating the names of God, in this case the name of Rām, everything is brought to completion, everything will be fulfilled.
>
> Repeating these names ripens our karma; the things that are not helpful for us are removed, and the things that are helpful for us are brought into the flow of our life—just through this practice, not through any action of our own. It's a ripening process.
>
> As we repeat these names over and over, the center of spiritual gravity deep inside us gets more solid, denser, and we're pulled

more deeply within ourselves. That gives us the ability, or rather creates the kind of conditions, to release a little sooner all the stuff that catches us in our minds and our emotions.

If you're thinking about something, whatever it is, say the weather, eventually that thought runs out of energy, right? It no longer holds you, your attention goes to something else and another thought takes you. Why should that process ever stop? Why should we ever come back to whatever place inside that we come back to?

In fact we are here, in our true nature; that's where we live. Our thoughts and our fascination with the external world and all the sensual and mental stuff and everything, that's what pulls us out of our true nature.

Through the repetition of these names we learn to sit more deeply in our own hearts. We become aware sooner that our mind is wandering. Little by little, gradually but inevitably, you enter more deeply into your own being, you recognize yourself in a new way.

Inevitably is an excellent word—*inevitably* means you're on a train, and the train is going one way, and you're at the front of the train running as fast as you can toward the back of the train, in the opposite direction from where the train is headed. But it doesn't matter, because when the train gets to the station, you get there too. That's *inevitably*. That's my life.

When you chant you don't have to imagine anything, have any fantastic experiences, visualize anything, or make anything happen. You're simply asked to sing, and when you notice that you're not paying attention, come back. That's all you have to do. There are no expectations you have to meet, which also means there's no disappointment. Don't expect a flaming chariot to come down from the sky and carry you away whenever you chant. It ain't gonna happen.

Just simply be here. When you notice you're not here, you already are! Then go back into the singing, with a little more intensity. Not trying harder, just giving it a little more attention. And then, as soon as you notice you've left again, come back.

Gradually, the fascination with external things wears away, the thoughts and emotions don't capture us as fiercely as they did, and the stories we tell ourselves about ourselves get less compelling. We begin to sit more deeply in ourselves and to find the Loving Presence within.

PILGRIMAGES

At the temple in India, we used to joke that Maharaj-ji's five-limbed yoga that we practiced consisted of eating, sleeping, drinking tea, gossiping, and walking about. It's true we were just hanging out, but we were hanging out in Maharaj-ji's presence at a temple in the Himalayas, in his vibratory space that was transforming us. We had traveled to the other side of the world to be there, some of us not knowing why or where we were going, but all searching for something within.

We might not have called it that at the time, but that was a pilgrimage. Perhaps a pilgrimage into our own hearts, but that is the best kind anyway. Later we experienced many other places in India that carry a spiritual charge, and we also found places in the West that have those qualities of deep peace and spiritual energy. If you're traveling or hanging out, you might consider making a pilgrimage to a holy site and using its spiritual energy as a way to intensify your own inner work.

RETREAT

A retreat takes you temporarily out of the profusion of sensory and mental input so you can concentrate on your inner life. Maybe all you have to do is close the door to your room and shut off the phone and the computer. On the other hand, you might consider a retreat at one of the many retreat centers in the West, where your aspirations are reinforced by other seekers, and where you can get pure food and some instruction in meditation or other practices. Listen inside for what type of retreat or center—whether it focuses on silent meditation or group chanting or some other form of practice—will work best for you and where you are in your journey.

WORDS FROM REALIZED BEINGS

Hanging out with realized beings or saints, with their words and pictures, is a way to inspire and find guidance for your own path. A realized being is like a pure mirror who shows you all of the places where there is dust on your own mirror. Such a being is a clear mirror because he or she doesn't have any attachments, so all you see are your own attachments writ large. Find words from the great saints and sages of the world's religions that inspire your practice. Copy them into your journal, put them on your refrigerator or by your computer, and take them into your heart. The words of realized beings have guided me over the years, and they will help you navigate your inner journey as they have mine. A few examples:

God, guru, and Self are One.
RAMANA MAHARSHI

The Self is the heart, self-luminous. Illumination arises from the heart and reaches the brain, which is the seat of the mind. The world is seen with the mind; so you see the world by the reflected light of the Self.
RAMANA MAHARSHI

The intense desire for God-realization is itself the way to it.
SRI ANANDAMAYI MA

Love has to spring spontaneously from within. It is in no way amenable to any form of inner or outer force. Love and coercion can never go together; but while love cannot be forced on anyone, it can be awakened through love itself. Love is essentially self-communicative. Those who do not have it catch it from those who have it. Those who receive love from others cannot be its recipients without giving a response which—in itself—is the nature of love. True love is unconquerable and irresistible. It goes on gathering power and spreading itself until eventually it transforms everyone it touches. Humanity will attain a new mode of being and life through the free and unhampered interplay of pure love from heart to heart.
MEHER BABA

Why is it so difficult to find God? Because you're looking for something you've never lost.
MEHER BABA

Knowledge and love of God are ultimately one and the same. There is no difference between pure knowledge and pure love.
SRI RAMAKRISHNA

A jar kept in water is full of water inside and outside. Similarly the soul immersed in God sees the all-pervading spirit within and without.
SRI RAMAKRISHNA

The saint is a mirror, everybody can look into it; it is our face that is distorted; not the mirror.
PALTU SAHIB

LISTENING TO YOUR SELF

Inner work can be subtle. As your mind quiets, you begin to listen more to your own inner voice. Learn to trust your own intuitive wisdom about your spiritual practice.

You can't buy someone else's judgments about your path; you can't buy a book's judgments. You have to run it through your own intuitive judgment. Maybe you say, "What I really need now is to develop a quiet meditative space, to quiet my mind more deeply." Or, "What I really need now is to open my heart." Or, "What I really need is a fierce teacher." Or "What I really need is a lot of loving, gentle support." Or, "What I really need to do is clean out my psychological stuff a little more before I can go on spiritually." If you really keep studying yourself, you will begin to feel where you are blocked and where your next turn in the path is. Trust it—learn how to trust your inner guide.

I'm a big advocate of the spiral path, of seeing spiritual work as a kind of spiral staircase. You may go very deeply into a practice, and if it starts not to work anymore, you pull back. Sometimes you do a practice for a while, then you go back into the world, or you try something else. When you come back to that practice on the next round, you see it from a whole new level. You see it from a different place in your consciousness. Who you are when you come back to it is different. So while a practice is a discipline, it's better to be gentle with yourself and not get too violent pushing yourself too hard. If you feel like you're getting ahead of yourself or starting to burn out, stop for a while and try other forms.

Some people come to me and say, "I think I ought to meditate," and I say, "Don't." Other people come and say, "Oh, thank God, I can meditate." It's just a matter of timing.

In our minds we often get ahead of our intuitive readiness in our lives or our being. We tend to overkill with our minds. We think our way into things; our mind conceives the next level of consciousness before we're really there or before we're ready to go there. The result is we're always a little ahead of ourselves in our thoughts. We don't slow down enough to be fully in our being. We're doing things as we *think* we ought to do them. We're constantly creating new models of ourselves before we're fully here with what is. If we can just slow down and be here now . . .

If you are doing a practice and the practice is not working, you listen intuitively inside, and you either hear, "If I reinvest in this practice and come at it from a new perspective, it could come alive in a new way," or "I'll go do something else for a while and come back to it again later on." You just have to trust however your intuition resonates in that moment.

My guidance is usually to go slow. Don't figure you're going to get enlightened yesterday. Relax. Just start to tune yourself to the spirit within. Don't make assumptions about how your path will go. You may say, "Finally, I've found my path, the practice that is right for me," but don't assume that practice is what you'll do for the rest of your life. Because the you who found that practice is, in the course of doing the practice, going to change into somebody else. A practice that was appropriate for you initially may not be useful further down the line. Keep staying open and hearing these delicate shifts and balances as they go on inside you.

There is value in deepening a practice. Swami Satchitananda once criticized me for being such an eclectic dilettante. He said, "Ram Dass, you can't just go around digging shallow wells everywhere. You have to dig a deep well so that you get fresh water." That's a good metaphor. I could come up with another metaphor that would be equally sweet for the other side of the argument.

But when I watch people over time, I see that they start out being very eclectic, trying different practices, then they get drawn into one practice quite deeply. When they come out the other end, like Ramakrishna, they can do all practices, and they're all the same. It's like a funnel or an hourglass: it all goes in one way through a narrow opening, and at the end it spreads out. So go gently. Allow yourself to keep trying things on and going into eclecticism until you genuinely feel pulled into a deeper process.

Gurdjieff, the Russian philosopher, said that while an alarm clock will wake you up at one moment, later on you may sleep right through it. You need to keep finding new alarm clocks to awaken yourself. He said you can have something that awakens you out of the sleepwalking of your normal waking consciousness that works one moment, but not the next. Like if you're reading something, you're reading it one moment, and a moment later you're busy planning your shopping list while you're reading it, and the next moment you've gone completely to sleep. Maharaj-ji once said to us, "The mind can travel a million miles in the blink of an eye. Buddha said that."

Practices are just practices. Practice makes perfect. Once you're perfected, practice is done. You use a boat to cross a river, but once you're on the other side, it's of no further use. At the level of pure being, there's nothing to do, but at the level of your ego, you want to do something. So do it. There's nothing to do, and yet you have to do it. You have to make the effort to practice, to do sadhana, but you also need to understand that the person who is making the effort never gets enlightened anyway. Understand that your ego who says, "Ooh, I can awaken," is ego that is going to die or disappear or dissolve in the process. Who gets enlightened is not who you *think* you are, but who you *are*. Finally, even your trying has to be given up.

Once I was sitting with the Tibetan teacher Chogyam Trungpa Rinpoche, and he said we would do this specific meditation on expanding outward. So we started to expand outward, looking into each other's eyes. After a while he said to me, "Ram Dass, are you trying?"

I said, "Oh yeah."

He said, "No, Ram Dass. Don't try, just expand."

There is this seeming paradox that exists between making effort and just allowing yourself to *be,* which are really two different planes of consciousness. When you, as an ego, sense there is something beyond your limited perception, you make an effort to go from A to B; you want to follow a path or take a journey. So you make the effort. You meditate. You go to a retreat. At first you may feel blocked and frustrated, so you force yourself; you discipline yourself. As the process works and you start to taste another level of awareness, you begin to see that those patterns of behavior, the trying and the frustration you experienced out of your desire for something else, were all within the cause-and-effect structure of your karma unfolding and how your mind works. In a sense, it was predictable. That you even seek to get enlightened or to get closer to God is a tendency (*sanskara* in Sanskrit) from your past actions that prepared you to now do spiritual practice.

There is a poignancy in our predicament of being stuck with one foot in the world and one foot in the spirit. When you get too holy or too high, the world pulls you back down. You have to dance with that kind of tension all the time. You keep bringing your worldly nature and your spiritual self closer and closer into alignment.

The good news is that awakening is built into the system. It just takes its own time. I've learned how to pump people up to experience a moment of awakening. Sometimes it's like having a tire with a big leak in it. You pump it all up, and then you turn around a moment later, and greed, lust, and fear have all returned, and it's flat again. You wonder what happened. Then with someone else, you just touch them, and they open; everything changes in their life, and they never go back. I'm learning to listen more carefully to who people are and where they are in their spiritual evolution. I'm learning to really honor people, and myself, for who we are in the moment, to understand the appropriateness of a practice and that our karma and our awakening are unfolding perfectly.

One of the greatest things that happened in my relationship with my father was when he was approaching death. I finally allowed him to be who he was instead of trying to make him into who I thought he should be. And he stopped trying to make me into who he thought I should be, and we became friends.

That's who we all are on this path, spiritual family and friends. It's just one big family. We're all relatives until we realize we're really all the same and there's only one of us—one loving awareness.

May you be one in that love.

Notes

CHAPTER 1

Page 3: "You never have to change what you see, only the way you see it."
Thaddeus Golas, *The Lazy Man's Guide to Enlightenment.* (Layton, UT:
Gibbs Smith, 2008) 89.

Page 3: "The mind can proceed only so far upon what it knows and can
prove ..." Albert Einstein, quoted in "Death of a Genius" by William
Miller, *Life* magazine, May 2, 1955, 64.

CHAPTER 2

Page 15: "The minute I heard my first love story ..." Rumi, *The Essential Rumi,*
translated by Coleman Barks with John Moyne. (San Francisco: Harper-
SanFrancisco, 1995) 106. Permission to reprint granted by the translator.

Page 21: "Devotion is easy and natural ..." Krishna Kumar Sah, "Bhakti"
(Malibu, CA: Love Serve Remember Foundation, 2011). Permission to
reprint granted by the author.

Page 24: "I will set You on my breath ..." Rumi, *Whispers of the Beloved,*
translated by Mafi Maryam and Azima Melita Kolin. (London:
Thorsons, 1999) 99.

Page 25: "My heart was split, and a flower appeared . . . " from "Odes of Solomon," *The Enlightened Heart: An Anthology of Sacred Poetry,* edited by Stephen Mitchell. (New York: Harper & Row, 1989) 24–25. Permission to reprint granted by the publisher.

Pages 17, 18: "Let me always feel you present ..." Psalm 19, "The Book of Psalms," *The Enlightened Heart: An Anthology of Sacred Poetry,* edited by Stephen Mitchell. (New York: Harper & Row, 1989). Permission to reprint granted by the publisher.

Pages 27, 28: "In his mind Hanuman had already crossed the sea ..." *Ramayana,* William Buck. (The Regents of the University of California: University of California Press, 2013). 182–184, 348–349. Permission to reprint granted by the publisher.

Page 29: "Hanuman, ever the humble servant, responds, 'Save me, save me from the tentacles of egoism!'" from Śrī Rāmacaritamānasa (Gorakhpur, India: Gita Press, n.d.), Descent V (Sundara Kānda), verse 32, 795.

CHAPTER 3

Page 35: "The Great Way is not difficult . . . " Seng-t'san, the third Chinese patriarch of Zen, *The Hsin Hsin Ming, Verses on the Faith-Mind* translated by Richard B. Clarke (Buffalo, NY: White Pine Press, 2001). Permission to reprint granted by the translator.

Page 41–44: "The train clanked and rattled through the suburbs of Tokyo ..." Terry Dobson, an American Aikido master (1937–1992), in "A Kind Word Turneth Away Wrath." This story has been widely reprinted and anthologized, but rights are unclear. It was said to have been printed in *Reader's Digest* in the 1970s and it is included in the anthology *The Awakened Warrior,* edited by Rick Fields (Tarcher, 1994) and in *Essential Spirituality* by Roger Walsh (John Wiley & Sons, 1999).

Page 59: "Are you looking for me? I am in the next seat ..." Kabir, from *Kabir: Ecstatic Poems* translated by Robert Bly. (Boston: Beacon Press, 2004). Permission to reprint granted by the publisher.

CHAPTER 4

Page 71: "I'd like to make more mistakes next time ..." Nadine Strain, from the poem "If I Had My Life to Live Over." This oft-reprinted essay is usually rendered as a poem, and the author's name given as Nadine Stair. But Kentucky journalist Byron Crawford, in his 1994 essay collection *Kentucky Stories,* writes that it was originally published as an essay in *Family Circle* magazine in March, 1978. The magazine misspelled the author's name: it should have been Nadine Strain. Strain was a resident of Louisville, Kentucky.

Page 74, 75: "Sometimes, ... I sat in my sunny doorway from sunrise till noon..." Henry David Thoreau, *Walden or, Life In The Woods* (Norwalk, CT: The Easton Press, 1981). 117–118.

Page 75: In a November 20, 1849, letter Thoreau wrote to Harrison Blake Concord, "I realized what the Orientals mean by contemplation and the forsaking of works. To some extent, and at rare intervals, even I am a yogi."

CHAPTER 5

Page 77: "But this: that one can contain ..." Rainer Maria Rilke, *Duino Elegies & The Sonnets to Orpheus,* edited and translated by Stephen Mitchell. (New York: Vintage Books, 1982, 1985, 2009) 27. Permission to reprint granted by the translator and publisher.

Page 79: "Don't prolong the past ..." Patrul Rinpoche from "On Meditation: Pithy and Powerful Words from Famed Teachers," *Shambhala Sun* magazine, March 2003.

Page 80: "Consider the possibility that the resistance to the pain and the fear pain may evoke ..." Stephen Levine, *Guided Meditations, Explorations and Healings* (New York: Anchor Books, 1991). Permission to reprint granted by the author.

Page 82: "Love and death are magnificent gifts, which many of us leave unopened." This line by Rilke is commonly translated as, "Love and death are the greatest gifts that are given to us, but mostly they are passed on unopened." In a personal communication, translator Stephen Mitchell told me, "I did some searching on the Internet and found this quote in German, though not the source: 'Die Liebe und der Tod sind grandiose Geschenke, die viele von uns ungeöffnet lassen.' The translation should say, 'Love and death are magnificent gifts, which many of us leave unopened.' Rilke doesn't say that they are *the* great gifts, and he doesn't say 'great'; nor does he say that we 'pass them on.' How could we pass on death? Death is given to us, not by us. The same for love. It's a gift that we *can't* pass on; we either open it or not, and that opening too is a gift. As is the not-opening."

Page 89: "Death is an illusion we all seem to buy into ..." Stephen Levine, *Guided Meditations, Explorations and Healings* (New York: Anchor Books, 1991). Permission to reprint granted by the author.

Page 85: "It may be argued that nobody can talk about death with authority who has not died..." Lama Anagorika Govinda in the foreword to *The Tibetan Book of the Dead,* compiled and edited by W.Y. Evans-Wentz (London: Oxford University Press, 1927). Permission to reprint granted by the publisher.

Page 91, 92: "Empty your mind of all thoughts ..." Lao-Tzu, #16 from *Tao Te Ching, A New English Version, with Foreword and Notes* translated by Stephen Mitchell (New York: HarperCollins, 1988). Permission to reprint granted by the publisher.

Page 94: "I am without form, without limit ..." Swami Rama Tirtha (1873-1906) from the poem "I am That." Accessed online.

CHAPTER 7

Page 113: "Since the day when I met with my Lord ..." Kabir, *One Hundred Poems of Kabir*, Poem XLI, I. 76. "Santo, sahaj samādh bhālī (O Sadhu! the simple union is the best)," translated by Rabindranath Tagore, (Madras: Macmillan & Co. Ltd., 1970) 48–49.

Page 121: "How did the rose ever open its heart ..." Hafiz, *Love Poems from God, Twelve Sacred Voices From The East and West,* translated by Daniel Ladinsky (New York: Penguin Compass, 2002) 161. Permission to reprint granted by the translator.

Page 122, 123 "Don't go outside your house to see flowers …" Kabir, from the poem "A Place to Sit," *Kabir: Ecstatic Poems* translated by Robert Bly (Boston: Beacon Press, 2004). Permission to reprint granted by the publisher.

CHAPTER 8

Page 132: "When you are with someone you love very much …" Swami Chetananda from *Songs from the Center of the Well*, (Portland, OR: Rudra Press, 1983). Permission to reprint granted by the author and The Movement Center, Inc.

Page 139: "People do not know what the Name of God can do …" Swami Ramdas, *Ramdas Speaks*, Vol 5. (Anandashram, Kerala: Bharatiya Vidya Bhavan, India).

Page 141: "Devotion to God who is seated in the hearts of us all is the one path …" Swami Ramdas, *Glimpses of Divine Vision*, (Mangalore, India: Sharada Press, 1944).

Page 141–143: "What we're singing is the repetition of the Divine Names …" Krishna Das, transcribed from a Maui retreat, December 2010. Permission to reprint granted by Krishna Das.

Page 144: "The Self is the heart, self-luminous …" Ramana Maharshi, *Maharshi's Gospel*, 13th ed. (Tiruvannamalai, India: Sri Ramanashram, 2002) 16.

Page 144: "The intense desire for God-realization is itself the way to it." Anandamayi Ma *Matri Darshan, Shri Anandamayi Ma*, translated by Atmananda Mangalam (Germany: Verlag S. Schang, 1983).

Page 145: "Knowledge and love of God are ultimately one and the same …" Sri Ramakrishna, *Ramakrishna: His Life and Sayings* by F. Max Müller (New Delhi: Rupa & Co., 2002) 138.

Page 145: "A jar kept in water is full of water inside and outside . . . ," Ibid, 141.

Page 145: "[T]he saint is a mirror …," Paltu Sahib, 19th century Indian saint from Ayodhya, quoted in *Sarmad* (Jewish Saint of India) by I.A. Ezekiel (Punjab, India: Radha Soami Satsang Beas, 1966).

Acknowledgments

JANAKI SANDY GAAL devotedly compiled material from Ram Dass's talks and writings before we knew this was a book. She was the original impetus for this project and helped at every step. She deserves vastly more credit than we can bestow.

Raghu Markus, director of the Love Serve Remember Foundation, approached Sounds True's publisher, Tami Simon, and chief editor, Jennifer Brown, with the idea of making an e-book, but they decided to go whole hog and bring it out in print. Sounds True's Amy Rost brought a life of editing expertise to bear on polishing *Polishing the Mirror*. She epitomizes the skill and enthusiasm of the Sounds True editing and production crew who have so beautifully midwifed and crafted this work.

Dassi Ma Kathleen Murphy kept the time and held the ground so this project could fly. K.K. Sah and Krishna Das contributed words from their individual journeys to our collective heart that reverberate with their affection. John Welshons lent a hand with a crucial, long-distance edit when he was providentially marooned on Maui by an East Coast blizzard.

Stephen Mitchell, Daniel Ladinsky, Richard Clarke, Coleman Barks, and Stephen Levine, among others, have been truly gracious in allowing their extraordinary work to be reproduced. The devotion and insight they bring to translating the great saints and poets, and the brilliance of their own expression, have enriched this text and the experience of working on it.

Spiritual books are but markers left beside the path for fellow pilgrims toward inner light. May dust from the feet of the great beings who have trod this Way before us grace the words and thoughts on these pages and guide us home.

About the Author and Coauthor

RAM DASS

Before becoming Ram Dass, he was Richard Alpert, son of the president of the New York, New Haven and Hartford railroad. Alpert was an up and coming professor of social relations at Harvard when he befriended a new faculty member named Timothy Leary. Leary had a transcendent experience with sacred mushrooms in Mexico, which he shared with Alpert. The two began a series of psychological research projects using substances that came to be known as "psychedelics." In 1963, they were fired from Harvard for pushing the limits with psychedelic research. From Ivy halls the duo went on to become counterculture icons, cresting the wave of the 60s.

By 1966 Alpert had taken psychedelic exploration as far as he could. He traveled to India looking for a map reader for the uncharted states of consciousness he had experienced. Through a seemingly fortuitous chain of events, he met a guru named Neem Karoli Baba, called simply Maharaj-ji, who *knew*. For six months Alpert lived a renunciate life in an ashram in the hills of the Himalayas. There he learned yoga and *bhakti* practice, the devotional path of the heart.

Alpert returned to America as Ram Dass, a name that means "servant of God." Feeling that he had brought back a precious jewel, Ram Dass began to share his experiences in talks everywhere and with young people who came to camp at his family's summer home in New Hampshire. At a commune in the mountains of northern New Mexico, some of his talks were transcribed and transformed into a spiritual tool box. It was published as a book in 1970. *Be Here Now* became a counterculture bible for millions of seekers setting out on a spiritual path.

Be Here Now resonated with a cultural moment in a way that few works have, before or since. Ram Dass continued to travel and lecture about spiritual work. For three decades his peripatetic life brought him in contact with thousands of individuals, and to collaborations with other teachers, like Chögyam Trungpa Rinpoche during the first summer of Naropa University. Ram Dass authored more books and helped start service organizations such as a prison ashram project, a project to help people die more consciously, and the Seva Foundation, which aims to cure blindness and serve less fortunate people around the world.

While in the middle of writing a book on conscious aging in 1997, titled *Still Here,* Ram Dass suffered a near-fatal stroke that left him with aphasia and paralysis on his right side. After a lengthy recovery, though wheelchair bound, he resumed traveling and lecturing—albeit more slowly. In 2004, Ram Dass traveled once again to India to visit Maharaj-ji's temple in the hills. When he returned to the States, he led a retreat on Maui, which ended with a trip to the emergency room due to a severe urinary and kidney infection. Once again, he nearly left his body. After the infection subsided, he settled on Maui. He no longer leaves Hawaii. Nowadays he teaches via the Internet on ramdass.org, leads retreats on Maui, and continues to write.

Since he stopped traveling, Ram Dass dwells in a quiet heart space. His signature teaching of just *being here now* has led to a level of deep contentment, and his accommodation of his physical limitation is as profound as his earlier verbal wit and wisdom were entertaining. Just as when he was a psychedelic pioneer probing new boundaries of consciousness, Ram Dass remains a trail blazer, now plumbing our spiritual heart for unconditional love.

RAMESHWAR DAS

Rameshwar Das met Ram Dass at a college talk in 1967 and went on to learn yoga and meditation from him at his family farm in New Hampshire. From 1970–72 Ramesh traveled to India to see Neem Karoli Baba. He still visits regularly.

Ramesh worked with Ram Dass on the 2010 book *Be Love Now*, on the *Love Serve Remember* recordings, and on the original toolbox project that became *Be Here Now*. He has also been a photographer, including a stint as a freelancer for the *New York Times* and other news publications. Ramesh's work spans a wide range of photojournalism, editorial, fine art, and commercial photography. He has taught photography and has also worked as an environmentalist and writer on coastal matters. He lives with his wife, a yoga teacher, on the east end of Long Island.

About Sounds True

SOUNDS TRUE is a multimedia publisher whose mission is to inspire and support personal transformation and spiritual awakening. Founded in 1985 and located in Boulder, Colorado, we work with many of the leading spiritual teachers, thinkers, healers, and visionary artists of our time. We strive with every title to preserve the essential "living wisdom" of the author or artist. It is our goal to create products that not only provide information to a reader or listener, but that also embody the quality of a wisdom transmission.

For those seeking genuine transformation, Sounds True is your trusted partner. At SoundsTrue.com you will find a wealth of free resources to support your journey, including exclusive weekly audio interviews, free downloads, interactive learning tools, and other special savings on all our titles.

To learn more, please visit SoundsTrue.com/bonus/free_gifts or call us toll free at 800-333-9185.

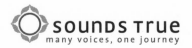